THE
WEIGH
DOWN
DIET

GWEN SHAMBLIN

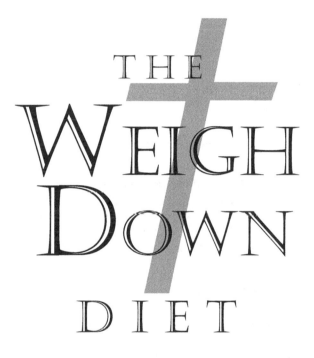

THE
WEIGH
DOWN
DIET

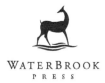

WATERBROOK
PRESS

THE WEIGH DOWN DIET
PUBLISHED BY WATERBROOK PRESS
12265 Oracle Boulevard, Suite 200
Colorado Springs, CO 80921

Trade Papaerback ISBN 978-0-385-49324-6

Originally published in hardcover by Doubleday in March 1997. Published in trade paperback in 2013 by Galilee, an imprint of Doubleday, a division of Random House LLC, New York, a Penguin Random House Company.

Published in the United States by WaterBrook Multnomah, an imprint of the Crown Publishing Group, a division of Random House LLC, New York, a Penguin Random House Company

The Library of Congress has cataloged the hardcover edition as follows:
Shamblin, Gwen.
The weigh down diet / Gwen Shamblin.—1st ed.
p. cm.
1. Weight loss—Religious aspects—Christianity. I. Title.
RM222.2.S467 1997
613.2'5—dc21 96–40222
CIP

Printed in the United States of America
2019

20 19 18

In memory of my father,
Walter Hodges Henley, M.D.,
March 24, 1927–Thanksgiving Day, 1981.
I remember him whistling as he made hospital rounds,
bowing low in prayer at church,
and confidently facing
death with peace.

And with loving thanks to my husband, David,
and to our children, Michael and Michelle.
Thank you for your patience, endurance,
and prayers during my writing.

Acknowledgments: I would also like to thank the staff at
The Weigh Down Workshop, especially the editorial team
that worked diligently together to make this happen.

TABLE OF CONTENTS

PHASE I

Phase II

INTRODUCTION

Welcome. You are about to embark on a unique program of weight reduction called the Weigh Down[†] Diet. This book gives you the major concepts of what is being taught in video and audio form in the Weigh Down Workshop[†] seminars across the country. Weigh Down[†] seminars are held in over ten thousand locations throughout the United States, Canada, and Europe, and are held in churches of all denominations.

We have entitled this book *The Weigh Down Diet*, but don't let the use of the word *diet* mislead you. The dictionary offers two definitions of the word diet. The first is "the food and drink regularly consumed." Another meaning is "to eat according to prescribed rules." We want to assure you that *The Weigh Down Diet* is founded on the complete freedom found in the first definition.

Weigh Down[†] is showing people, on a daily basis, how our God can transform their hearts and minds so that they can rise above the magnetic pull of the refrigerator! Instead of emphasizing the caloric content of food, the Weigh Down Workshop[†] encourages you to focus on your natural, internal hunger control. But more importantly, your focus will be trained to turn toward the will of God as it relates to food!

Studies show that we are fatter than ever. And it seems that the more weight-obsessed we are, the less we lose and the more we revile the pudgy, the plump, the rotund, the fat, and the morbidly obese. The billion-dollar weight-loss industry is a dizzying carousel of promises, hardly ever fulfilled.

Years of restrictive dieting have only strengthened the chains of slavery to food. Years of focusing on food and giving all our boredom, distress, and troubles to a pan of brownies have only increased our stress. Dieting has drained us emotionally, if not financially, and has exacerbated rather than solved our problems.

Into this vortex comes the Weigh Down Workshop[t], which can offer up testimonials as enthusiastic as anything television weight-loss gurus or liquid fasts ever produced—the inspiring sagas of women and men and children who lost 20, 50, 180 pounds and counting.

Chapter after chapter, this book will guide you away from dieting—which we define as "making the food behave." If you are dieting, taking pills, counting fat grams, using exchange lists, or changing the content of foods, then you believe your basic problem is the food. Weigh Down[t] counters this by maintaining that dieting keeps the person focused on what he or she should and should not eat. This focus on food only increases the magnetic pull of the refrigerator. This book emphasizes God's power—not "will-power."

If you are willing, the journey you are about to take will be a magnificent wisdom-gaining experience, rescuing you from dieting and taking you to permanent weight loss.

In the end, it wasn't the low-carbohydrate diet or local weight-loss groups that helped thousands lose the nagging extra pounds in a matter of months—it was God.

Do not care what people think-do not consider how big or little you are—do not think of yourself at all. If God puts this course of action on your heart, then come along. God does not call perfect people; He calls imperfect people to be devoted to Him so that we can see His awesome and mighty right hand rescue us!

Through much devotion to our true God, the Lord Almighty,

Gwen Shamblin
Founder, The Weigh Down Workshop[t]

MEDICAL CONSIDERATIONS

Before starting this program, we recommend that you receive a medical checkup. Consulting your physician is especially vital if you have any medical condition which is impacted by food/foods.

You are preparing to move into the realm of "regular foods" from the grocery store, including things with salt and fat and sugar. However, your volume of foods is going to be drastically reduced, and your body loves this! God made us sensitive to what and how much our bodies need, and you have to resurrect this system!

If you have preexisting health conditions such as food allergies, diverticulitis, cirrhosis of the liver, diabetes, hyperlipoproteinemia, bowel resections, chronic ulcers, kidney disease, chronic constipation, etc., make sure that you are under your physician's care and guidelines for foods and medication. For example, if you have chronic constipation, you must keep eating your fiber. If you have ulcers, take your medicine and do not eat the foods that upset your stomach.

However, there are a few preexisting physical conditions that may be alleviated when you lose weight and start eating regular foods in smaller amounts. For example, if you have high cholesterol or triglycerides, losing weight permanently could possibly alleviate this problem. You must stay in touch with your physician. Spastic colon and ulcers could slowly improve as you eat the volume of food that your body calls for. PMS symptoms are often less intense as you lose weight. Joint and muscle problems are improved in some cases. People on cortisone and/or who have lupus will still lose weight with no problem—it just might be a slower weight loss.

When I take medication which should be taken with food, I take it with one to three crackers. Consult your physician.

You are not going to believe how much energy and life you are going to enjoy, as well as how much emotional improvement you will experience!

Type I and type II diabetes and hypoglycemia

Consult your physician and make sure he or she is fully aware of the principles of this program.

Type I diabetics need to know how to check their glucose levels regularly and to adjust insulin intake accordingly as the volume of food decreases. They must eat when their blood sugar is too low and when they feel hunger.

Type II diabetes (adult-onset) is usually the direct result of over-eating. The body is overburdened by the ingestion of too much food, and the pancreas is unable to produce enough insulin to handle the excess. Diabetics who have come through the program have some-times been able to regulate their insulin level and eliminate medication by simply reducing their intake of food, which gets the insulin/food ratio closer.

Occasionally, low blood sugar and hunger do not coincide. If blood sugar levels drop, do not panic! Usually, small amounts of food taken within a few minutes will make you feel better. This is not an open invitation to binge.

Children

This book is written addressing the overweight adult. Information on overweight children and eating practices for children may be found in Appendix B

PHASE I
HOW TO BECOME A THIN EATER

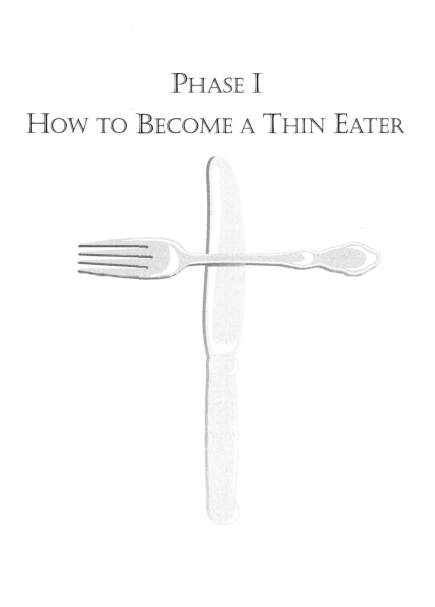

THE WEIGH DOWN APPROACH
What does God have to do with this, anyway?

W*ith God's help* you *can* learn to stop in the middle of a meal and have no desire to eat the second half if your stomach is satisfied! God did not put chocolate or lasagna or real blue cheese dressing on earth to torture us, but rather for our enjoyment. However, He wants us to learn how to rise above the magnetic pull of the refrigerator so that food does not consume our lives!

The problem and the solution

We have been created with two empty, needing-to-be-fed holes in our body. One is the stomach, and the other is the heart.

The *stomach* is a literal hole in our body which is to be fed with the proper amount of food. As for the *heart*, I am speaking figuratively of our deep-down feelings. To satisfy these deep-down

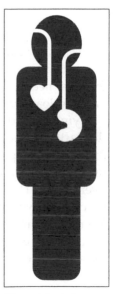

Figure 1-1: God created two empty places in each of us.

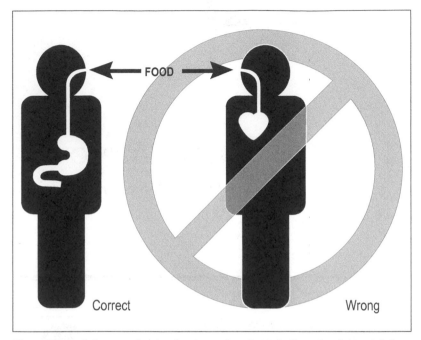

Figure 1-2: Feed the stomach only when it growls and stop feeding when it is satisfied (not stuffed). Using food to fill the heart leads to overweight.

feelings, needs, or desires of the heart, we may often turn to food and overload our stomach with more than it needs.

Trying to feed a hurting, needy heart with food or anything on this earth (alcohol, tobacco, antidepressants, sexual lusts, money, the praise of other people, etc.) is a common error. The person who attempts to feed a longing heart with food will stay on the path to overweight. Those who pursue an overindulgence of alcohol or tobacco or power will also reap the consequences of those pursuits. There is nothing inherently evil about food, alcohol, tobacco, money, credit cards, etc. However, it is wrong to become a slave to any of these things or to let them master you.

The solution for overweight

As you can see from the diagram, we have been trying to feed our hurting, longing hearts with physical food. We have also learned to love food. Therefore, the solution is as follows:

1. Relearn how to feed the stomach only when it is truly hungry.
2. Relearn how to feed or nourish the longing human soul with a relationship with God.
3. Relearn how to recognize the different "hunger" urges and not confuse them.

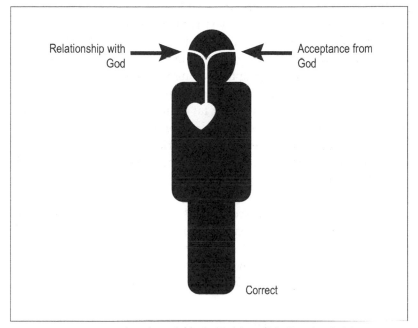

Relationship with God →   ← Acceptance from God

Correct

Figure 1-3: Our heart and needs are fed by looking for and finding that God is our Financier, Comforter, Mechanic, Lawyer, Physician, Counselor, Friend, Husband, Defender, Trusting Leader, and Father.

Am I a failure?

Your major concerns will be: "How can this work for me? Because:

1. "I feel a distance between God and me because I thought He made me overweight and, for years, has not answered my prayers to take this weight off."
2. "I've tried every diet five times, every diet pill and exercise, and failed miserably—so how can this work?"

What we are really asking is... "Am I a failure, or is God angry at me and sabotaging me?"

Well, you are not a failure, it is not genetic, and God is not sabotaging you. He does hope that your slavery to diets and overweight will make you call out to Him. He is in love with you, and He wants you to depend on Him for deliverance so you can see how mighty He is and how important you are to Him.

Why have diets not worked so far? The reason is that you (like me and the rest of the world) have tried using man-made rules (diets) instead of God's rules. God has never asked anyone to eat food off of a list, to count fat exchanges, or to take an appetite suppressant. You have just been applying the wrong medicine to this condition. You were using your willpower and man's rules. God is too smart to let a local weight-loss group or fat gram counting be your *Savior* and thereby get all the credit. Man-made rules will not work.

Now, welcome to the Weigh Down Workshop†, a place that teaches you God's rules for eating and shows you the futility of man-made rules. Welcome to the Weigh Down Workshop†, a place that shows you how to use God's strength rather than your willpower! Welcome to the Weigh Down Workshop†, a place where thousands of people are now thin after years of trying.

In summary: *you are not a failure.* You have been using man's rules and your willpower, and now you are going to use God's plan for eating and His strength. There is hope, and God will get the credit!

Diets will never work

Diets do not get to the root of the problem. In fact, diets aggravate the problem rather than alleviate it. Diets just boil down to making the food behave. Food companies have spent several decades and millions of dollars to pull out the fat and calories so that the food is righteous! Actually, billions of dollars are spent by the food industry to make us feel needy. Many food companies may not want us to succeed in losing weight, but, rather, would prefer to make us feel dependent on them so we will consume whatever is sold. In fact, the more diets fail, the better off the industry is.

The root of the problem is not the food ingredients, but how much volume is going down the old hatch (our esophagus)! And, indeed, we consumers have wanted the food industry to take the fat out of the Twinkie so that we can simply eat more Twinkies. Changing the food but not changing the volume of what is swallowed will leave us on a roller coaster of weight loss and weight gain. Changing our metabolism or our nervous system by taking pills and hormones is not permanent, because we cannot stay on them because of the side effects. The motivation to be thin is not vanity—it is natural. God has programmed us to want the best for our bodies.

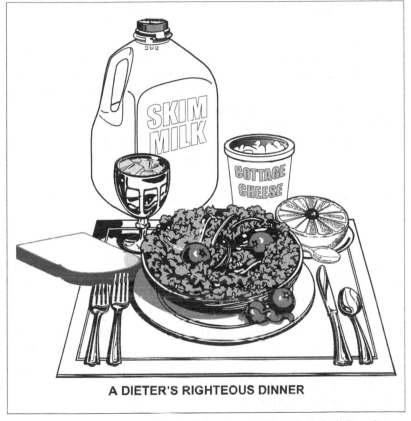

A DIETER'S RIGHTEOUS DINNER

Figure 1-4: Diets have encouraged eating large volumes of low-calorie food. Once dieters go off the diet, they have become accustomed to the large volumes. They gain their weight back and blame the food. We must rethink this. It is not the food-it is being accustomed to large volumes of food!

We cannot continue to have the doctor suck out the fat from one part of the body (suction-assisted lipectomies) while we continue to stuff our mouths. We must surrender the root of the problem; that is so much easier to do than diets or surgery. Weigh Down[t] is different from all other diet systems because it is not selling a diet plan, a food, or whatever. It is selling a future, a future to be filled and fulfilled. Hunger is filled, God's love is embraced and enjoyed, and appetites are under control and given to God.

Do you have to be religious to do the program?

For those of you who do not feel particularly religious—do not worry. You have exactly what you need to be able to do this program. You see, each of us has a heart to worship, and we all adore something. That tells us we have the capacity to give our heart to something. The question is: can you transfer your devotion from one thing to another? The answer is: *yes!*

Giving our hearts over to something is a learned process and can be relearned. For example, some people *enjoy* sports, but other people seem to *worship* sports. Some people enjoy material things, but other people seem to worship things. Some people use money, but other people will do anything to get it.

Some people use food for fuel to run the body, and some people dream about food. Some of these dreamers have been known to get up in the morning and find the bony remains of fried chicken on their chest! This old relationship with food can be transferred to a relationship with God or to a heart for God.

In the past you may have loved the feeling of planning a binge and dreaming over recipes, cookbooks, and magazines that have food plans and pictures of food. You may have looked forward to the feeling of waiting for everyone to go to bed (and they had better not get back up out of bed) so you could prepare, cook, and consume the food without the judgment of anybody.

The good news is that you can relearn how to get that feeling from the Lord. When you learn to get this happy feeling from finding God, you will experience much more fulfillment. Bingeing out on seeking God has no yucky, guilty, depressing side effects. In other words, it is possible to let go of that old way of having fun and re-place it with something so much more filling (yet with no calories!). By choosing this new path you will lose weight and never regain the weight.

I know some of you are reading in disbelief. I can hear you think-ing, "You're telling me that if I am not hungry and want to eat a pan of brownies, that I should go to the Bible and read it instead!?" This concept is not "pie in the sky." Keep reading. I dare you to let me prove this to you.

Thousands of people have taken the Weigh Down Workshop[†] seminar or have read this book. They no longer get this "binge high" from food, but from focusing completely on our true Heavenly Fa-ther and trying to please Him. Jesus said, "My food is to do the will of Him who sent me and to finish His work" (John 4:34).

Some people have experienced a "high" when they became in-volved in exercise. While the "high" is not wrong, it is not complete. And usually, obsessive, tedious exercise to become thin eventually *wears* thin if the exercise is self-focused rather than God-focused. Exercise, like food, must also be put in its place and not worshiped, but enjoyed.

The transfer to a heavenly focus from a focus on food, exercise, or anything else is much more delightful and fulfilling. It has so many rewards that you will never want to return to giving your heart to anything else!

How do you lose weight?

Once you stop going to food for sensual indulgence, escape, spac-ing out, a tranquilizing effect, comfort, and so on, and start swal-lowing regular foods only when your stomach growls, you will swal-low or eat just one-half to one-third of what you used to swallow. The *desire eating* goes away. That means you will lose weight! You will be able to do this; it happens naturally. You will not have to measure the food or count the grams—your stomach will guide you. The volume of food decreases as you focus on hunger and fullness. Thousands of ex-dieters are doing this within twenty-four hours of starting Weigh Down[†].

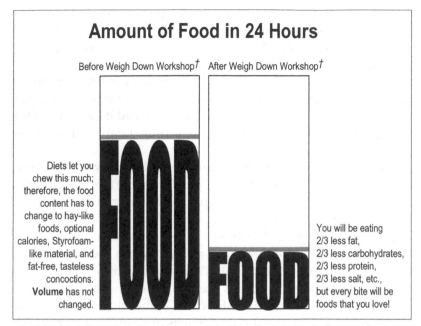

Figure 1-5: Expect your food consumption to go down in this program—anywhere from one-half to two-thirds.

The typical weight-loss program suggests losing weight through diet and exercise. We suggest that if you lose the passion for food, the result will be that you eat less food and therefore lose weight permanently. The typical 1950s-1990s approach tried to fix the body or the food but did not address the passion. The Weigh Down Workshop† approach fixes the heart first, and the body follows.

We are not running against the current national medical suggestion that the fat content needs to be reduced; rather, we just propose another means to accomplish this goal. The Weigh Down Workshop† will show you how God can bring us to peace with food—never to return to the nightmare of endless overweight, yo-yo dieting and "have-to" exercise regimens, but rather to a calm, nonmagnetized approach to regular foods with the ability to approach foods such as rich entrees and desserts without losing control. Exercise need no longer be connected to burning calories; instead it can be an enjoyable activity. You will be free!

Before | After

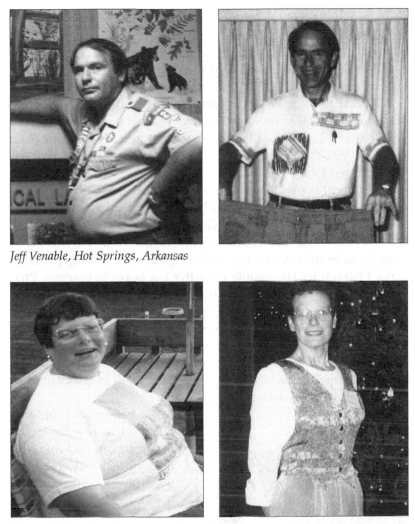

Jeff Venable, Hot Springs, Arkansas

Virginia Schnacky, Bloomington, Minnesota

Notice that people who follow the principles of the Weigh Down Workshop† have learned to eat less food and have become happy with eating less food! In other words, these people are happy and full of something else. We will explore this "something else" throughout the book.

What to expect on the journey

You are about to embark on a unique program of weight reduction. Instead of emphasizing the caloric content of food, our focus will be on your natural, internal hunger control; more importantly, our focus will be trained to turn toward the will of God and away from a focus on foods.

We liken the journey you are about to take—from the slavery of diet programs (fat gram and calorie counting) and overweight to being a normal eater—to the journey the children of Israel took from the slavery of Egypt, through the Desert of Testing, and finally to the Promised Land.

The Biblical book of Exodus in the Old Testament is the age-old story of the exodus of God's children from Egyptian bondage. Do you remember the story of how God parted the Red Sea? God sent Moses to lead the Israelites and to let them know that He was delivering them from bondage. God sent plagues upon the Egyptians to make Pharaoh let His people go. After ten horrible plagues, Pharaoh let the Israelites pack their bags and go. Pharaoh changed his mind and tried to recapture the Israelites, but God parted the Red Sea with a mighty east wind. Once the Israelites were safely on the other side, Pharaoh's mightiest warriors and finest chariots and horses were buried by the sea as God put the water back into its place. The Israelites had witnessed God's mighty deliverance of them from the clutching hands of Pharaoh.

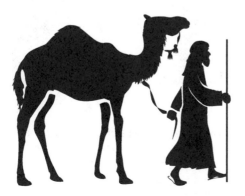

But before God could let His children inherit the Promised Land flowing with milk and honey, He took them on a journey through the Desert of Testing. Deuteronomy 8:2,3 says, "Remember how the LORD your God led you all the way in the desert these forty years, to humble you and to test you in order to know what was in your heart, whether or not you would keep his commands. He humbled you, causing you to hunger and then feeding you with manna, which neither you nor your fathers had known, to teach you that man does not live on bread alone but on every word that comes from the mouth of the LORD."

Just like the Israelites, you will experience a deliverance from dieting and the bondage of food and diet programs that treat you like children. This book will explain to you how thousands have handled the Desert of Testing. Finally, you will be shown how to follow in the footsteps of God's children who entered the Promised Land of milk and honey. "So if the Son sets you free, you will be free indeed" (John 8:36). The Promised Land is a place out of the hot Desert of Testing, a place where you no longer feel tempted to eat when your stomach is not hungry.

No matter what your age, no matter what your size, no matter what your means of control— whether it be dieting, exercising to keep the weight off, bulimia (vomiting the food to maintain control), anorexia (extreme bodily deprivation for means of control), or just flat giving up self-control, this program is for you.

As recorded in the Bible, God came to rescue His people, the Israelites, from slavery. He got the old and the young, the bricklayers and the basket weavers, the weary and the brokenhearted. God came, and He rescued them all.

You are about to read how thousands have turned toward God and watched Him rescue them from the love of food and, therefore, the unwanted pounds. There is hope for you, for it is by no coincidence that you picked up this book.

You will ultimately find that God has *everything* to do with weight control!

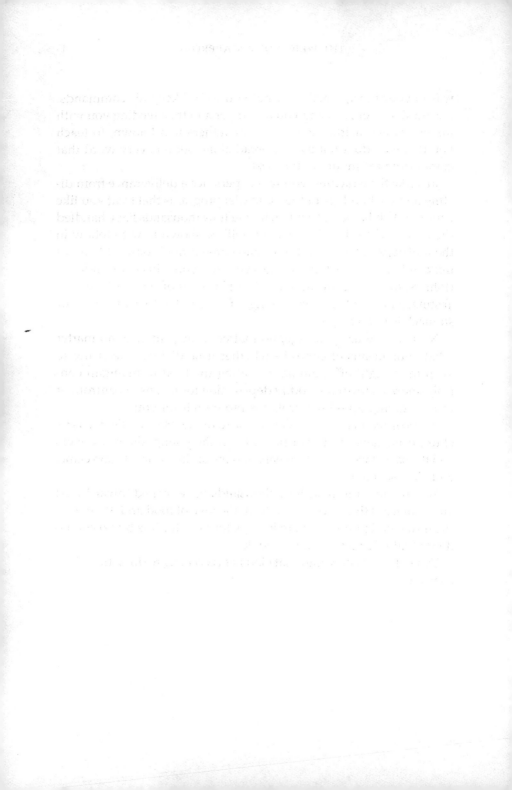

THE STORY OF WEIGH DOWN

I was a thin eater growing up. I can remember my father saying that my eyes were bigger than my stomach as I selected more food in the cafeteria line than I could eat. This was possibly more of a good stewardship lesson than a health lesson on my father's part, since there were four children to feed. At that point in my life, the pain of overeating made more of an impact on my eating than the pleasure of indulging the taste buds. Nevertheless, it revealed the beginnings of a tiny seed of greed for food. Had the seed of greed been redirected, it could have saved me years of grief.

My mother was a member of the clean-your-plate club, as were all good American mothers who came out of the Great Depression. We were highly indoctrinated to good foods and bad foods. Fruits and vegetables were righteous items in our household. This combination of approaches to foods was backed up in schools as gospel, and the Basic Four food groups were memorized as national government teachings. I can remember getting stars if I "cleaned" my plate at school in third grade. This combination of teaching, that is still taught today—as right as it may seem—has helped to unplug the God-programmed internal hunger and internal ability to select foods (a natural biological feedback to cue the body to a variety of foods).

As I entered the teen years, the pain of overstuffing lessened. My father had been correct at one time about my eyes being bigger than my stomach—but by now, after years of strengthening the stomach and freely feeding my *head hunger,* my stomach could easily accommodate my eyes! Besides the increasing greed, fear was already a part of my life. There were four children in our family, and if I did not "get mine," there might not be any left. I felt that I had to look out for myself. I was older and freer to make my own food selections, and I had not been trained even to consider true stomach hunger and fullness. I quickly crept up five to ten pounds. The problem with even five excess pounds on my body type is that it all went to my waist and not to the area of my body that was in dire need of some extra meat—my legs! Since my body would not cooperate with me by evenly distributing my weight, even five pounds overweight really distracted me, since most clothing stores did not make things to fit potatoes with toothpick legs.

My father had been correct at one time about my eyes being bigger than my stomach—but by now, after years of strengthening the stomach and freely feeding my head hunger, my stomach could easily accommodate my eyes!

Thank goodness I loved cheerleading. The inner drive to be a good cheerleader kept me jumping around for years. Apparently, I was overeating approximately the amount of energy I was expending. In other words, my exercise was disguising or at least compensating for my overeating. Once cheerleading ended and college began, my overeating was unveiled in the form of extra pounds.

Moreover, the University of Tennessee sold what I called "magic cards" that allowed students to go to the cafeteria of the generous state university from 7 o'clock in the morning to 7 o'clock in the evening. At any time of day, we could serve ourselves milk shakes, soft drinks, ice cream and shelves of desserts. Breakfast overlapped lunch, which overlapped supper. The foods were fantastic, and all you needed to enter this massive all-you-can eat cafeteria was the magic card. It was magic because we paid a onetime fee at the beginning of the semester, which gave us unlimited privileges.

After 7 P.M., when the megacafeteria closed, the campus delicatessens came alive. The smell of the steamed fresh sandwiches with melted cheese called my name every night. Well, the result of the combination of no more cheerleading and increased exposure to volumes of foods (without my mother around to correct me) was another ten pounds.

I was now ranging from ten to twenty pounds over my pre-college weight, and all of the fat was around my waist. Now, instead of a potato with toothpick legs, the new look was a pregnant potato with toothpick legs! I was becoming desperate. But my mere physical twenty pounds overweight did not reveal how deeply food-focused I was. I knew no end to fullness, and I tried throwing up my food after a binge but was not coordinated enough. The endless cycle of diets/exercise and weight loss/weight gain was deeply entrenched by now. I loved to eat and eat and eat. Although it felt good to stuff myself, I felt enslaved. As lightly or as humorously as I might describe this out-of-control situation, in reality, it was a very insecure time for me.

The undergraduate degree I was working on was in dietetics, and my graduate study was nutrition science. Unfortunately, these degrees only increased my wayward focus on food and self. I wondered if I had every malnutrition-related disease that the books covered. I tried the exchange diets the nutrition books recommended, and after a few years of failure, I started trying everything in the back of the book that was listed as "unreliable weight loss methods," such as the low carbohydrate diets that put the body into ketosis (a self-inflicted, temporary diabetic state). At the university, I enrolled in aerobics classes that used unsuccessful, questionable techniques to motivate college students to lose weight. One class actually had us contract to lose weight for a grade. I was in a cocky mood and contracted or agreed to lose fifteen pounds for an "A." I made a "C" in that class, which meant not even the highly valued grades could make me lose weight. I could not get this stuff off my body!

The most common diet regimen I used looked something like this: morning was starvation; noon was lettuce, Italian dressing, and a diet soda; and in the evening I allowed myself a few exchanges. I would then try to jog on the tracks at night. I could tolerate this regimen until Thursday night, but the thought of the fun planned for the weekend would always tempt me into "letting go." Once I was "off" of my diet—watch out. I would mix up a batch of cookie dough and eat much of the raw batter as well as the baked. I never had a lot of confidence that exchange lists would work for me because I was so good at cheating. For instance, usually by Tuesday I had borrowed all the fats and carbohydrates for the entire week, and by Thursday I had eaten most of the optional calories allowed for the month!

I started to feel like a failure for the first time in my life, and that started affecting other areas of my life.

The whole situation seemed hopeless, especially during evening temptations. At 9 o'clock at night when everyone else was eating a Shelbourne Towers famous kielbasa deli sandwich with smoked cheddar cheese, Claussen pickle, chips, and a diet soda, I would look on my sheet of paper and see that all I had left was a fruit exchange. I did not want fruit! Proponents of exchange lists would always say, "All you have to do is move the exchanges over, and when you are done for the day, you are through!" Wrong! That is when the problem begins. Temptations such as these seemed to make me graze through the whole kitchen for anything but fruit.

The ever-vigilant scales always told the truth of my wasted efforts. I had netted no weight loss. I was getting nowhere! But I refused to acknowledge defeat and would use my own strength to start over again on Monday morning on the same regime with hopes that I could pull it off this time. It was baffling me, since I seemed to be fairly successful at other things in my life. Why couldn't I do this? I started to feel that something was wrong with me. I started to feel like a failure for the first time in my life, and that started affecting other areas of my life.

Somehow, in my degree studies, I saw that virtually none of the experts saw fit to mention our Creator. This made me suspicious of some of the theories that were being offered in dietetics. I just did not buy the idea that all overweight was a result of genetics or was inherited. Making the food behave by dieting did not add up, either. It never explained how my grandparents were at their right weight while eating bacon and eggs every day. In fact, they had never heard of light cream cheese and skim milk. They had the best of the best coconut cakes, homemade ice cream, and pecan pies. Fried chicken and bread and butter were not condemned. Food was enjoyed, and diets and exercise were never a part of the conversation. We had delightful "real" foods at my grandmother's house and great grandparents' houses, and all were at their ideal weights—all except me, the highly educated dietetics student and professional dieter.

My studies kept me up-to-date on efforts to change the food content and on the dangers of too much fat and too much sugar. We touched the edge of behavioral approaches to weight loss, and I felt as if that was much closer to the answer than the study of food content. However, parking my car in a more distant parking lot and putting my fork down between bites did not stop the desire in my heart to continue chewing through the refrigerator and pantry contents at 10 o'clock at night when no one was looking. Behavior modification techniques were not the answer, either!

A friend who lived in the apartment next to me was skinny—very skinny. I decided to interview her. Why have skinny people not been a resource for overweight people over the years?

There are several reasons. Thin people have learned to avoid threatening conversations that start off asking, "How come you are so skinny?" or "How can you eat chocolate pie and not gain weight?" Skinny people are well aware of their unpopular position in life. They are also aware that they are doomed no matter what answer they give. If they have bought the genetic or inherited theories and answer, "I guess God just made me this way," that would insinuate that God just made the fat person fat! That is like signing their own death warrant, and if not, that answer is likely to cost them a friendship. If they answer, "Well, I don't know. I guess I eat less food than you do," they have again threatened the friendship. So they politely answer, "I don't know, and I never see you eat anything." And then they quickly change the subject.

Therefore, since I knew that I would get nowhere by asking any questions, I asked my skinny friend if I could just watch her and write down what she ate in the next forty-eight hours. (By the way, this is your first assignment—to watch someone eat who does not diet or exercise for weight loss and has been thin all his life.) The first eating occasion she had for the day was at noon at McDonald's. I had already eaten my whole Big Mac, large fries, and milk shake, and I was nursing a diet drink. She was still working on the first half of a quarter-pound hamburger! Then she did something strange: she started to rewrap the second half of her hamburger. I was astounded. I tried asking her what she was doing. She said, "I don't want any more." So I asked the next obvious questions: "Are you sick?" and "Are you sure you are from this planet?" She said that she was not sick and that she was from Tennessee.

My thin-eating friend was never able to tell me why she could stop in the middle of the hamburger. That untold secret was going to prove to be the missing key to the great mystery of permanent weight loss.

I asked her to please tell me what she was thinking. How could she throw away food from McDonald's? You see, not only could I eat my Big Mac, large fries, and milk shake, but I could eat her Quarter Pounder as well. And I really wanted the food from the people at the table next to me, but I was too polite to ask for it. As I said before, I knew no end to fullness. I was never satisfied; I had lost the ability to feel pain from being too full. My heart and soul cried out for more. Ephesians 4:19 described my situation: "Having lost all sensitivity, they have given themselves over to sensuality so as to indulge in every kind of impurity, with a continual lust for more."

My thin-eating friend was never able to tell me why she could stop in the middle of the hamburger. That untold secret was going to prove to be the missing key to the great mystery of permanent weight loss. Within any forty-eight hour period, my skinny friend did not eat as much as I ate. She might have eaten a lot at one meal and then skipped the next one. Over the entire period, she ate smaller amounts of food.

I just started imitating this fascinating behavior she displayed—not knowing how I was doing it. I lost my excess weight in 1977 and married the following year. By 1980, I had my first child. I had eaten everything that I was hungry for, but *only* when I was hungry. I gained fifty pounds at least and had a ten-pound, twenty-three-inch baby boy, Michael, who scored a perfect ten on the Apgar index. He was beautiful. I ate only when I was hungry and lost all my weight within a few months, back to 105–110 pounds. I could not believe it. I gained forty-five pounds with my second pregnancy, and I had an eight-pound baby girl, Michelle. In the eighth month of my third pregnancy, I lost my baby boy, Matthew, to unknown causes. Even under heavy sorrow, I knew Matthew was being raised by the Father. I went to God for comfort—not food—therefore, I lost all my weight again. I was really on to something, but what—I was not sure.

In the midst of pregnancies, in 1982, I decided to open up my home for the first twelve ladies at church who wanted to work on their weight. Being so ingrained in dietetics, I tried a combination of diet, exercise, behavior modification and an introduction to hunger and fullness. I was open to any suggestions. This was the beginning of many years of mistakes and failures and rare success, if you defined success as I did: success is having no desire to overeat again. In fact, success would be the feeling that overeating is repulsive.

By 1986, I had eliminated what I believed did not work and had a body of knowledge of what I believed did work. I could educate people on how to get the weight off, but aiding them in *keeping* the weight off was the problem. I realized that I could stop in the middle of a hamburger and I, like my friend back in college, still did not know how in the world I did it. I also knew that I would never be overweight again. How could others experience this? So I prayed to God for wisdom. The scriptures and understanding started coming in little by little, and I started incorporating this into the original Weigh Down Workshop* counseling center.

What happened as a result of a more God-focused workshop was phenomenal. We knew that the information should not be just for a select few; many people believed that the workshop could be held in churches or small groups. I prayed for God's guidance, and God really blessed this idea. In less than five years, the Weigh Down Workshop[†] is in ten thousand churches and small groups throughout the United States, Canada and Europe. The statistics of the weight loss are almost impossible to measure because it has grown so quickly. But we know that the reason Weigh Down Workshop[†] has grown quickly is because the weight loss results are phenomenal— in other words, the statistics are great! The letters and the phone calls include testimonies of how a focus on God can turn people's lives 180 degrees. These testimonies are wonderful, and our office sees and hears them daily. We will share some of them later in this book.

After praying to God for wisdom, the answer to *how* I was able to permanently lose weight became clearer and clearer. So now we have a new definition of weight loss success. It is not defined by weight loss, because anyone can lose weight. Rather, weight loss success means losing both the weight and the desire to overeat. Once you lose the desire to binge or overeat, you never gain back the excess pounds.

What took years for me to learn will unfold over the next few chapters. You need to know that I lost my weight, never to go back to a focus on food or a desire to eat the second half of the candy bar if my stomach was full. And that is one great statistic.

AN UPDATE ON THE
PROFESSIONAL DIETER

I f you look back in the archives of history, you will see that people have been altering their food content and taking pills to lose weight for quite some time. Being overweight is not a new problem. In fact, the Bible records that one of Israel's high priests, Eli, was "heavy." He lived about 1100 B.C. Over the years, the study of food, its contents, and its health benefits have been topics of great interest.

In my years of working with people who have weight problems, no one has ever asked me to help them become overweight, and yet people of every race and creed, even if they are five pounds overweight, ask for help with getting the weight off. I concluded that God made all people to desire to be at their right weight and that this is not greedy or vain, but rather, a healthy, innate drive programmed in us by God.

Nutrition, as we know it today, is a very young science. The first "dietitian" on record was in the early 1900s. By 1945, scientists had been able to identify, isolate, and duplicate the chemical structure of a vitamin. By the 1950s, our medicine cabinets were beginning to be dotted with vitamin concoctions—something our grandparents never consumed, yet they still lived long enough to be grandparents. The early human nutritional discoveries were wonderful, but perhaps they sparked a tiny flame of more trust in science than in the Creator of science—God. Some people suspected the Bible was obsolete. Many of us behaved as if we, too, believed that Jesus did not realize what our lipid profiles and medical charts would look like in the 20th century when we read Mark 7:14–23:

> Again Jesus called the crowd to him and said, "Listen to me, everyone, and understand this. Nothing outside a man can make him 'unclean' by going into him. Rather, it is what comes out of a man that makes him 'unclean.' " After he had left the crowd and entered the house, his disciples asked him about this parable. "Are you so dull?" he asked. "Don't you see that nothing that enters a man from the outside can make him 'unclean'? For it doesn't go into his heart but into his stomach, and then out of his body." In saying this, Jesus declared all foods "clean." He went on: "What comes out of a man is what makes him 'unclean.' For from within, out of men's hearts, come evil thoughts, sexual immorality, theft, murder, adultery, greed, malice, deceit, lewdness, envy, slander, arrogance and folly. All these evils come from inside and make a man 'unclean.' "

Was God no longer necessary now that we had educated men and honorable educational institutions? Had God gifted the 20th century physicians, scientists, nutritionists, and dietitians so we would consult them rather than bother Him? Never mind the scripture that reads, "In the thirty-ninth year of his reign Asa was afflicted with a disease in his feet. Though his disease was severe, even in his illness he did not seek help from the LORD, but only from the physicians. Then in the forty-first year of his reign Asa died and rested with his fathers" (2 Chronicles 16:12–13).

The mid-twentieth century brought an attitude that it is useless to turn to God for advice about good health. Some people began to doubt that God had already set up most healthy body processes and natural healing processes. These attitudes went hand-in-hand with the belief that individuals are responsible for analyzing the caloric and nutritional content of everything edible and for relating this knowledge to the complicated needs of the human body.

We became suspicious of every grocery store and every "processed" food (whatever that means, since everything we eat has to be processed in some manner to get it into our house). This new mindset turned into a blazing fire of distrust of eating regular foods found in the grocery store. We now had tackle boxes full of vitamin pills.

So Scripture such as "Do not worry about what you eat or drink" was long forgotten and replaced with an obsession of worry about missing nutrients and about our human body and its needs. As the population became more focused on food and our physical bodies, the population—especially in America—continued to get heavier. There seemed to be a connection.

By the 1970s, the health promotion movement hit an all-time high, and so did our concern for maximum nutrition and meeting one hundred percent of the U.S. RDA (United States Recommended Daily Allowance). We were trying to eat less, but we were *Weight loss support groups began to spring up in virtually every neighborhood. In the meantime, the population gained even more weight.* so afraid of missing nutritious foods or a key nutrient that we ended up overeating and finding ourselves heavier. Weight loss support groups began to spring up in virtually every neighborhood. In the meantime, the population gained even more weight.

The Metropolitan Life Height & Weight Tables, which are nothing more than updated statistics from the latest mortality data, continued to set the average weight per height up another few pounds, so that even if we netted an extra five-pound weight gain every five years, we were still in the "normal" category.

By the 1980s, most of us dieters had become professional dieters, since we utilized exchange lists and attended support groups an average of three to ten times a year. Many could tell the carbohydrate, protein, and fat content, as well as the total calories, of every food on the market. Most professional dieters could tell how much energy was expended when walking up the steps, vacuuming the house, and mowing the lawn, and we knew every free food or optional calorie available to the consumer. There were exercise aerobics classes on every corner. If it was Monday, and we were in the right mood, we would slap down another registration fee and take home our sheet of foods we could eat and foods we could not eat. We were at it again, because maybe this time it would work. It was almost like the slot machine in Las Vegas. If we put another quarter in, maybe this time it would pay off!

The search for "healthy foods" continued, resulting in millions of people focused on their health, almost as if a person could add a single hour to the life that God allotted him. Job 14:5 says, "Man's days are determined; you have decreed the number of his months and have set limits he cannot exceed." And Matthew 6:27 says, "Who of you by worrying can add a single hour to his life?"

During early Bible times, people often lived longer than today's average of seventy-two to seventy-five years. And they lived this long without help from dietitians or current nutritional prompting. Take a look at this scripture referring to people who lived thousands of years ago. "Then the LORD said, 'My Spirit will not contend with man forever, for he is mortal; his days will be a hundred and twenty years' " (Genesis 6:3). God shortened the life span to 120 years. Please keep in mind that we are well aware that you could possibly play a part in shortening your life. For instance, you could try to commit suicide or indulge too heavily in tobacco, food, alcohol or drugs. But you have also heard of people who tried to commit suicide but whose efforts did not work. As you may know, overweight is the single most related factor to early death, even though we all know of exceptional cases of obese people, like the high priest Eli, who lived until they were ninety. *God* is in control.

By the 1980s, many dieters had experimented with every diet pill—whether over-the-counter, prescription, or even, unfortunately, under-the-counter. As the population continued to gain weight, the number of weight loss methods exploded and the price for weight loss increased. It was possible to spend three thousand dollars for supervised liquid protein diets with hopes that the more we spent, the more we could shift responsibility for success to the people in the white coats. Surely, for a higher wage, we could depend on that outside force to make the increasingly less-motivated professional dieter stay on the program. The secret dream of the professional dieter was to go away to a fat farm and come back transformed. The farm staff did everything for us—plan, cook, clean up—we just paid them to do it for us. Many of us found ourselves going to hospitals for stomach stapling and suction-assisted lipectomies. Yet the population as a whole continued to gain weight.

In spite of our using more professional health-care givers and spending more money, the results were disastrous. Hope was disappearing as our weight was at an all-time high. Even loving and motivational weight-loss gurus could not talk us into one more diet, and we emptied our pocketbooks on the painful (and questionable) surgical and liquid diet procedures. Exercise became an all-time popular means of keeping weight down, but like the cookie with less fat being offered to the public, it was talked about and considered, but not realistically adopted by most of the population. We could not logically fit exercise time into our schedules, nor could we out-exercise our over-eating. Much of the population that did try to adopt exercise moved from slavery to fat grams to the locked-in feeling of *having* to exercise or put fifteen pounds back the minute they stopped. Slavery again!

And the population lost fifteen pounds—but gained another twenty pounds.

In the early 1990s, with no new solution on the market, the desperate, overweight population started doing things that expressed defeat. The white flag was waving in the air. The defeated professional dieters who had already tried to make the food content change were now trying to get the world to change: make the airplane seats larger; make the oversized clothes more beautiful and acceptable; make the bus aisles wider; make the food even lower in fat. And the subtle but most telling underlying change wanted by the professional dieter was the attitude of others: "The people around me are now going to have to like me as fat, because that is exactly how I'm going to stay!" "We cannot lose weight; therefore, to be able to handle the pain of this situation, we are going to try to get people to accept us as we are." But down deep, people knew this was not the answer either, because God has programmed the heart of mankind to desire that the body should be at its right weight, and the health problems that follow overweight and obesity continue to reinforce this longing. We could get our spouse to "shut up," but down deep, they would prefer us to be thin.

So here we are today, heading into the 21st century. Hope is gone and anger toward life, fellow man (especially nauseatingly skinny people) and even God has set in. If this describes where you are with your professional dieting career, then believe it or not, you are not alone. Instead of feeling defeated and hopeless, you can have great hope. These years of dieting have not gone to waste. Rather, they have deeply ingrained in your heart that diets do not work permanently. Everything that has happened to you has been used to plow up the soil and bring you to the planting and harvesting stage in your life.

Those who read this book now are in the "broken state"—the state of heart and mind that does the *very best* with the Weigh Down Workshop†. You should expect great results as you become a thin eater. It does not surprise me that we had to exhaust every available weight loss method created by man before we would finally ask God to help.

Once again, God is the genius of behavior modification. He programs us to long for this correct weight and the good knee joints and circulation that go with it, and He does not reward band-aid approaches to these problems.

The Weigh Down Workshop† will prove to be a very refreshing approach to the weight loss dilemma—a journey away from professional dieting and the worry that you are missing a vitamin. Your energy will be restored much like that of a fish put back into the water. This approach will differ greatly from the energy-draining battle of forcing down another salad or piece of skinless chicken. Turning to God will be the major missing key to permanent weight loss. But what does it mean to turn to God, and how do we tap into His resources? Have we not all cried out to God to take the fat away? Hang in there. The answer is just ahead . . . .

WHY DIETS DON'T WORK

and Why You Are Not a Failure

Before we begin learning the new approach, I want you to know why diets do not work. This will help explain why you have not been successful and give you more hope that *you* are not a failure and that you can do this program.

Diets do not work because they are basically just making the food behave. When we have taken out the sugar and replaced it with an artificial sugar, thrown out the fat and replaced it with an artificial fat, thrown out the calories and replaced them with non-caloric fluff or indigestible hay, we have made the food behave or change. We have not changed our own behavior. We do not have to change how much food we chew and swallow, because the food itself has changed to larger volumes of low-calorie content. One

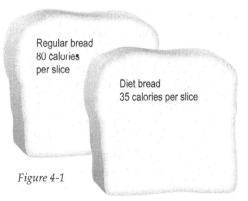

Regular bread
80 calories
per slice

Diet bread
35 calories per slice

Figure 4-1

serving piece of food that used to contain 115 calories now contains only 70 calories. Since the same volume of food now contains fewer calories, you can eat a larger volume. Never mind that it is tasteless and unpalatable. You do not have to take fewer bites of food to lose weight; you can even take more bites on a diet. However, you eventually go back to the regular foods. This is inevitable because you get sick and tired of diet food, and your body craves regular food. As a result, you gain weight back quickly because you were reprogrammed to chew even more food while on the diet!

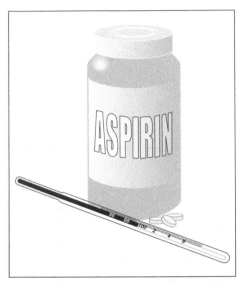

Figure 4-2: Aspirin does not get to the root of the bacterial infection. Likewise, diets do not get to the root of overeating.

Pills, liquid fasts, appetite suppressants, and counting fat grams change your environment temporarily, but they do not change you. They are like taking aspirin for a fever. Yes, the fever goes down temporarily, but as soon as the aspirin wears off, the fever goes back up. Why? It is because the aspirin does not get to the root of the problem—the bacterial infection. What you need is an antibiotic.

We believe the Weigh Down Workshop* approach is the antibiotic or what is needed to get to the root of the real problem. The real problem can be partially defined as a desire to put more food down the esophagus than the body wants or, put another way, wanting to chew more food than the body can handle. Making the food behave by changing its content (low fat, low calorie) will not help you change this desire to chew more food. In fact, dieting is the perfect environment to cultivate a deeper love for food. Using the Weigh Down Workshop* approach, we will not ask the food to behave. Instead, we will teach *you* how to behave. More importantly, we will teach you how God can take away the desire to overeat.

Just as dieting does not help your heart desire less food, neither does exercise. Exercise has virtue for physical training. There is no substitute for exercise when it comes to muscle toning, cardiovascular conditioning, and bone strengthening. It can also help with digestion and with healthy functioning of your organs. "For physical training is of some value, but godliness has value for all things, holding promise for both the present life and the life to come" (1 Timothy 4:8). *We believe that exercise is great for physical training, but it does not retrain your over-chewing.* Exercise could even work against you in terms of weight loss. Our goal is getting you to chew less food. But it is very tempting to continue to overeat and then compensate by walking around the block. Do not misinterpret—we are all for exercise. However, our goal is to focus all of your heart, soul, mind, and *strength* on eating less food. The only exercises we insist on are getting down on your knees to pray and getting the muscle of your will to surrender some of the extra food you have been eating. That is a whole new exercise. (Many are too large to get on your knees right now. That is OK—just get on your knees in your heart.)

> The only exercises we insist on are getting down on your knees to pray and getting the muscle of your will to surrender some of the extra food you have been eating.

Just know that everyone who traveled this journey and lost weight permanently did not have to increase energy expenditure through exercise. Not everyone can exercise. What about the disabled? What about the person who loves to exercise but has been injured? Are these people doomed to gain weight? *No.* Let me explain.

Exercise will not increase the speed of your weight loss, because you now will be using hunger and fullness as your signals to eat. In exercise, your body needs more oxygen, so immediately and automatically, you breathe harder. Exercise will also make you more thirsty. You will require more water to satisfy your body's needs, so you will automatically drink more water until those needs are met. Likewise, even though hunger is deferred temporarily, within twenty-four hours, your body's hunger increases automatically to cover the body's extra caloric needs. So if you want to exercise, fine; but exercise will not help you to lose weight faster. It will allow you to eat more food, just as it allows you to drink more water. The goal of the Weigh Down Workshop† will be a decreased *desire* to eat large volumes of food. If you are less active because of an inability to exercise, your hunger will decrease to meet your fuel needs. You never have to fear missing an aerobics class or workout again.

The body was made perfectly—you will be learning to listen to it and trust God's programmed signals.

A scripture from the book of Colossians is one of the first I found that applied to the problem. These few verses were the beginning of some foundational verses that grounded the Weigh Down Workshop†, and that would be used to unravel the mystery. Let us look at Colossians 2:16 and 20–23:

> Therefore do not let anyone judge you by what you eat or drink
> . . . Since you died with Christ to the basic principles of this world,
> why, as though you still belonged to it, do you submit to its rules:
> "Do not handle! Do not taste! Do not touch!"? These are all des-
> tined to perish with use, because they are based on human com-
> mands and teachings. Such regulations indeed have an appear-
> ance of wisdom, with their self-imposed worship, their false
> humility and their harsh treatment of the body, but they lack
> any value in restraining sensual indulgence.

The passage above is mainly a discussion of man-made rules versus God's rules. What does God really want for mankind? When God had called His dear children out of Egypt and set them apart so they would be distinguished from other nations as pure, holy, rich, and blessed, He gave them separate food rules. These rules were not only to make them unique, but they were to symbolize that, to be in God's presence, they were to be clean. The external cleanliness symbolized that the heart was to be clean.

When Jesus came to Earth, He explained that, prior to His arrival, the outside had to be clean. But now the use of external cleanliness to symbolize cleanliness of the heart is de-emphasized because Jesus has made it possible for us to actually be clean on the inside. Now God can be near us without the food rules. Jesus set us free from those tedious rules. Even without them, we can enter the Most Holy Place—God's presence.

Let us examine the passage in Colossians 2, starting with verse 16: "Therefore, do not let anyone judge you by what you eat or drink."

Simply put, you are free. Stop judging yourself for desiring and eating dessert in public. Likewise, stop judging others who are eating rich sauces and fat-filled meats! God has set us free from the food rules. Remember, Jesus described God as a father who would kill a fatted calf for the return of a prodigal son (Luke 15:11–32)! So who are we to judge? God did not accidentally leave the Basic Four food groups out of the Bible!

God did not accidentally leave the Basic Four food groups out of the Bible!

Remember the words of Jesus in Mark 7:14b–20: " 'Listen to me, everyone, and understand this. Nothing outside a man can make him "unclean" by going into him. Rather, it is what comes out of a man that makes him "unclean." After he had left the crowd and entered the house, his disciples asked him about this parable. 'Are you so dull?' He asked. 'Don't you see that nothing that enters a man from the outside can make him "unclean"? For it doesn't go into his heart but into his stomach, and then out of his body.' In saying this, Jesus declared all foods 'clean.' He went on: 'What comes out of a man is what makes him "unclean." ' "

It is not what is outside of a man that makes him right or wrong, clean or unclean, righteous before God or a sinner—it is what is in the heart of man. Continuing with Colossians 2, resuming our examination at verse 20: "Since you died with Christ to the basic principles of this world, why, as though you still belonged to it, do you submit to its rules: 'Do not handle! Do not taste! Do not touch!'? These are all destined to perish with use, because they are based on human commands and teachings" (Colossians 2:20–22).

This is just a continuation of verse 16, a continuation of the liberation from dietary rules by Jesus and an admonition to look for God's will instead of man's rules. So you are going down the right path if you do not let people judge you, but rather you look for God's judgment and what He wants. You are going down the right path if you follow Jesus Christ, who has just come from the Father and knows

It seems so right to count fat grams, but doing so never stops the heart from wanting more!

exactly what God considers important and unimportant. You are doing a good thing if you are examining the rules you go by in your life. It is good to consider which of them are simply man-made rules and not God's ideas at all. Diets do not work, because they are man's rules. Man's rules may change the environment around you (as the content of the food may change), but God's rules change the heart of mankind. God will thwart man's rules so that we do not worship man, and He will make His rules work beautifully so we will be drawn to His genius and power.

Now let us look at verse 23: "Such regulations indeed have an appearance of wisdom, with their self-imposed worship, their false humility and their harsh treatment of the body . . . ."

As long as you are feeling self-righteous about eating diet foods, then you are missing out once again. It is a false humility and a self-imposed worship, so you are missing out on true worship. It is tricky because man-made rules have an appearance of wisdom. It seems so right to count fat grams, but doing so never stops the heart from wanting more!

The reference to the harsh treatment of the body—at the end of this verse—is a valid point. When you go by man-made rules, such as diet rules—eating large volumes of low-calorie foods is one of the man-made rules—you could possibly develop spastic colon, indigestion, dumping syndrome (diarrhea), and other conditions that irritate the body and make you feel uncomfortable.

Verse 23 contains the first key to unlocking the mystery: ". . . but they lack any value in restraining sensual *indulgence*." Have all these man-made rules done anything to make you less attracted to the magnetic pull of the refrigerator? Would you agree that the opposite is true? After dieting for a couple of decades, have you become even more focused on food than you were before, and have you found it even more difficult to diet or restrain your eating?

We can conclude that the more we diet, the more we focus on ourselves. This can prove to be a bad focus, as it gets us nowhere but feeling sorry for ourselves, which usually plunges us deeper into depression. In addition to focusing on ourselves, diet rules also make us focus on food. We get up in the morning thinking about what we are going to eat and what we are not going to eat. We allow ourselves to indulge, so to speak, our lust toward craving food. If we have been doing that for very many years, we realize that we can actually become enslaved to this lust which, again, is trying to feed that longing heart.

To sum up the verses: God does not care about *what* we eat. Do not let others judge us, and do not feel self-righteous about following those man-made rules. What God does care about is *how much we eat*. God cares about and is displeased with overindulgence.

These verses set the stage for the Weigh Down Workshop[†] foundational points, which are as follows:

- *Stop dieting for two major reasons.* First, it makes you focus on yourself and your body. Second, it makes you focus on food. The more you focus on planning, buying, preparing, cooking, serving and eating the food, the stronger the magnetic pull to the refrigerator. In other words, dieting provides the perfect setup to accelerate your love for food.

- *Do not focus on what people think.* Stop allowing people to judge you when you are eating pecan pie or regular foods of any kind. Every time you find yourself wondering what people think, turn your attention straight upward to God and look only for His approval. Similarly, stop feeling self-righteous when you have pulled the fat out of a recipe and made the food behave. It is time to relearn how to be righteous (do things God's way) by making your mouth behave.

- *Stop feeling like a failure.* You have not overcome overeating because you have applied the wrong medicine to this condition. It is time to start over with new hope. You can change your heart's focus.

• *Understand that this behavior you are tackling is overindulgence.*
Overindulgence leads a person to desire something on this *earth*
to make him feel good. Our loving God will give you this feeling
so that you no longer have to look for it from things on this earth.
It is time to direct that desire upward toward God to let Him fill
you, for what you are hungering and thirsting for is God. Another
key to unlocking the mystery of permanent weight control: making
the food behave will not work. Admitting we need to behave, with
God's help, is the beginning of the end of overweight!

IT'S NOT GENETICS
OR YOUR MOTHER'S FAULT

It is no wonder we cannot get to the root of some of the problems in our lives. Over the last few decades, some professionals
have labeled many of our behaviors as chronic conditions.
Granted, many of the problems in our lives really are diseases. Wonderfully advanced medical procedures and protocols can alleviate
true physical problems. We praise God for His opening up great
minds to advanced medical practices for conditions out of our control.

But we need to question the people who label some of our behaviors with long, technical terms. When they label a self-willed behavior as a disease—or worse, a chronic or terminal-sounding condition—then many of us are programmed to believe we need hospitals, white-coated medical professionals, prescription drugs, and
special concoctions. Once you have been labeled as bulimic, anorexic, or obese, and then read current theories that you are genetically overweight, you could really feel trapped. Who could muster
up the energy to combat chronic genetic obesity, bulimia, or anorexia nervosa that is genetic or inherited?

Another thing that could make you feel hopeless is counselors

informing you that you have come from a "dysfunctional family."
Well, who has not come from a dysfunctional family!? Look at the
first family unit: Adam, Eve, Cain, and Abel. Cain killed Abel by
knocking him on the head with a rock. Every family or person has
problems, and sin is in all lives and in all families. You are not alone,
and your situation is not hopeless. I believe God when He speaks
through the Apostle Paul: "No temptation has seized you except
what is common to man. And God is
faithful; he will not let you be tempted

There is hope, my
friends . . . You are
not a failure—your
family is not a fail-
ure and your genes
are not sabotaged.
Your problem is not
physiological, psy-
chological, congeni-
tal or inherited.

beyond what you can bear. But when
you are tempted, he will also provide
a way out so that you can stand up
under it" (1 Corinthians 10:13).

There is a way out, friends! And do
not try to shock me with your family
background story or your present horrible marriage situation or your physical condition.

I have seen married forty-five-year-
old women lose over a hundred
pounds.

Women diagnosed with lupus or
kidney disease lose weight while under heavy doses of cortisone.

So do men who claim terrible marriage situations or who have
terminally ill children to care for.

People on the verge of bankruptcy, who have had no job offer for
over twelve months, lose weight.

So do insulin-dependent diabetics and people confined to wheel-
chairs.

Women lose weight who have lost a parent or child, or who are
heavily depressed because they have moved away from everyone
they know.

So do women and men diagnosed with cancer.

Even lonely teenagers who have had to live with the pain of being made fun of daily have lost over a hundred pounds.

On the opposite end, I have seen people diagnosed with anorexia and bulimia who have not had more episodes.

Life is bittersweet for us all. Personally, I lost weight after each pregnancy. I lost my baby in the eighth month of my third pregnancy, and even under heavy sorrow, I lost all my excess weight with God's help.

Why do we look for theories that suggest genetics or our dysfunctional family triggered our overeating or bizarre eating habits? Well, such theories do temporarily make us feel better about the overweight condition we are in, but, after the temporary good feeling wears off, they leave us depressed, and with no hope.

There *is* hope, my friends. There is great hope for you. You are not a failure—your family is not a failure, and your genes are not sabotaged. Your problem is not physiological, psychological, congenital, or inherited. You have a wonderful opportunity to make a choice to eat less food, and we will show you how to do that in the next chapter.

God has great plans to prosper you and return all the years the locusts have eaten.

"I will repay you for the years the locusts have eaten —
    the great locust and the young locust,
    the other locusts and the locust swarm —
    my great army that I sent among you.
You will have plenty to eat, until you are full,
    and you will praise the name of the LORD your God,
    who has worked wonders for you;
    never again will my people be shamed.
Then you will know that I am in Israel,
    that I am the LORD your God,
    and that there is no other;
    never again will my people be shamed." (Joel 2:25–27)

Come with Him now out of Egypt into the Desert of Testing—a place for just you and God alone. There, you will find out that He is your everything—that nothing else will really matter anymore.

How to Feed the Stomach

To relearn how to feed the stomach, you first need to wait for true stomach hunger. The stomach is a pouch made out of three layers of muscle, and it is located right below your sternum bone—the bone that is broken open in heart bypass operations.

This feeling of true stomach hunger we are looking for is a little burning, empty, hollow sensation that occurs several hours after the last feeding (or *many* hours after the last binge!). It is a very tiny, polite feeling, and I have known novices in Weigh Down Work-

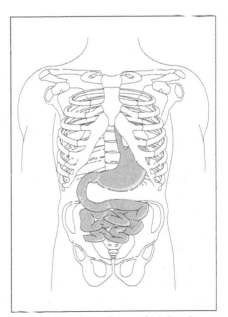

Figure 6-1: Position of stomach under rib cage

shop[t] seminars to pass it by or give it antacids, thinking it was indigestion!

You can pray to God to help you recognize true physiological hunger. You will discover that His prodding is normally gentle. He is trying to wake us up to His leading rather than dictate to us. God projects many images of Himself; I see Him as a kind shepherd and a gentle man. "Come to me, all you who are weary and burdened, and I will give you rest. Take my yoke upon you and learn from me, for I am gentle and humble in heart, and you will find rest for your souls. For my yoke is easy and my burden is light" (Matthew 11:28–30). That is why hunger is only a polite nudge and why you need to be a little more quiet, still, and calm to find this rumbling of acid underneath the ribs. Some people feel this burning at the waistline; some feel it up in the esophagus. No matter. If you are not sure that this feeling is hunger, just wait a little longer.

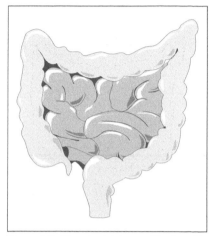

Figure 6-2: Do not mistake rumbles from the lower intestine for stomach growl.

Remember, you will always feel great while you are waiting! Many Weigh Down Workshop[t] participants wait for a growl or rumbling in this pouch. Disregard the rare rumblings and noises that originate below the belt line or where the belt line used to be. That is just the noise of trying to digest the "last supper." Those noises from the lower intestine are the sounds of the digestion of food you ate a few hours previously.

Before the end of this chapter, you will know how to tell if you are truly physiologically hungry. To start with, do not be afraid to wait a few hours for hunger; you will feel great. Jesus went to the desert and fasted forty days. We are not suggesting that you do this; however, throughout history a fast of a few days has been reported to be a good thing. There are many examples of people fasting (bypass-

ing hunger), but we are only asking you to wait for—not bypass—
your first hunger signal. This is not a fast. This is normal behavior.

Note: See the special notes for diabetics and hypoglycemics starting on page 59.

How to eat

Waiting for stomach hunger
will be like waiting for the "E"
(empty) on the automobile fuel
gauge. Your normal blood sugar
after a meal ranges from 80 to
120 milligrams per deciliters of
blood. When your blood sugar
level drops to eighty milligrams
per hundred deciliters of blood,
the hypothalamus (a part of the
brain) senses this drop. The
brain then sends a message by

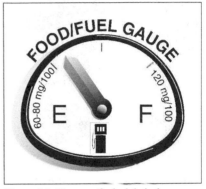

Figure 6-3: Hunger: the body's fuel gauge

means of hormones and nerve impulses to the stomach to produce
hydrochloric acid, which, in turn produces an empty, hollow, burning, hunger sensation. Your stomach was designed to make and
handle this acid production. Acid production, digestion, and absorption of food are all controlled by your nerves (central nervous system) and hormones.

The difference between you and a car is that your body has stored
fuel (your fat stores) so that you really do not run out of gas. It should
not be scary to go to empty "E"; rather, you should welcome it, for
this is how you will lose your excess weight. Your body, in its awareness of having an excess of stored fuel, will burn that stored fuel
(stored as body fat) if you eat the amount that the body calls for.
Eventually, you will return to your ideal body weight. If you reach
this state of hunger and cannot get to food, within ten to twenty
minutes the body will pull a meal from your hips or gut and send
these fat stores into the bloodstream. The result—the hunger growl
goes away and you have fuel to run on.

However, you are not to ignore the growl. That would be as wrong

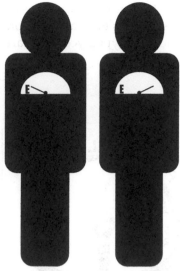

Figure 6-4.

as ignoring the full signal to stop. Let go of control and obey the body, making reasonable exceptions for special situations we will discuss later.

Do not refuel before you reach hunger. You will have more energy and time than you have ever had while waiting for hunger. When your blood sugar drops—this is normal—the stomach walls produce hydrochloric acid, which makes the stomach growl or feel empty. This is your signal to eat. It is healthy to empty out or not to eat until hungry.

We suggest that you drink only noncaloric drinks—such as water, diet sodas, and artificially sweetened tea—while you are learning how to sense the body's needs. If you drink sugared tea, milk, fruit juice, sports drinks, or regular soft drinks throughout the day, the glucose (sugar) from them will keep your blood sugar up, the result being somewhat like an I.V. bag in the hospital. If the blood sugar levels stay elevated, then the stomach will not growl or feel hungry.

You will sense a clearer stomach signal while drinking only noncaloric drinks. Continually popping mints or hard candy, chewing sugared gum, and taking cream in your coffee will have the same effect on blood sugar. All of these things will keep your blood sugar level up and possibly keep you from sensing hunger. However, feel free to eat or drink whatever you want within the context of hunger. If you are having a meal and want sugared tea with it, that is fine.

Drinking sugared and naturally sweetened drinks (juice) is the number one reason that children do not want to eat or do not want solid foods and some-times become anemic. Limit sweet drinks and start using noncaloric drinks or water. Water is the stuff people take baths in—but in most U.S. locations, you *can* drink it straight from the tap; it does not require an extra filter on the faucet or have to be the bottled variety.

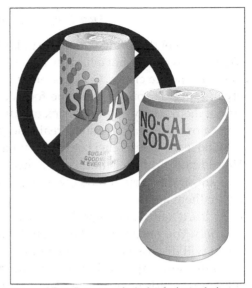

It is our experience that it would be better for you to stop drinking sugared drinks and transfer over to noncaloric drinks. It takes approximately three

Figure 6-5: Select non-caloric drinks instead of sugary beverages or sports drinks between hunger or eating occasions.

weeks to switch over your taste buds from regular pop to noncaloric soda. Going back to the old drink will taste weird after three or four weeks. It is easy after the third day if you do not go back and forth. You can train your taste buds to like anything! God programs us to naturally like what we get used to. Perhaps variety is good for the body, up to a point.

Another suggestion: do not feel that you *must* drink eight glasses of water per day. That is an old diet rule that can actually make you sick. Overconsumption of water causes *hypernatremia,* a word that means "too much water in the bloodstream." Symptoms include diz-ziness and nausea. You might have seen hypernatremia in infants who were made to swim; they got sick from swallowing too much water. Remember, anything in excess is not good for you, including water. Use your thirst mechanism; it keeps you perfectly balanced. Try to stop guzzling from sixty-four-ounce thirst busters. Trust your breathing mechanism, sleep mechanism, thirst mechanism, and your hunger mechanism. God has made them to work perfectly.

How to approach food

Once you feel this hunger, select regular foods that you desire. The foods you want are not evil. This includes pizza, Fritos, sour cream, desserts and ice cream. God has programmed you to desire a variety of foods. If you eat the same foods over and over, you will get sick of them. Many of you are sick of skinless chicken or salads with low-calorie dressing. Try some real blue cheese dressing. It is fantastic! God is the genius chef behind lasagna and chocolate cheesecake. He did not put bagels and cream cheese on earth to torture us! If you are sick of certain foods, you are free to avoid them until you desire them again. That is a very healthy nutritional practice. Your body has a natural biological feedback mechanism that cues you to a variety. You need to trust how your body was made. In later chapters, I will discuss how this low volume of regular foods is a superior nutritional approach, and it is the diet regime that almost all ninety-year-olds have always followed. In other words, it is associated with good health.

But for right now—please trust me—know that no one following Weigh Down Workshop[†] principles has died from scurvy, beriberi, pellagra, or any other disease associated with nutritional deficiencies.

When you get hungry, think about what food you would like. Be reasonable. If what you are craving is at a restaurant halfway across town, sometimes God has granted you the time and money to be this picky; but if not, please settle for the next best thing.

I will give you an example: I am hungry right now—I feel empty.

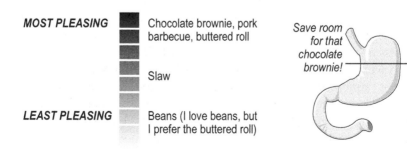

MOST PLEASING — Chocolate brownie, pork barbecue, buttered roll

Slaw

LEAST PLEASING — Beans (I love beans, but I prefer the buttered roll)

Save room for that chocolate brownie!

Figure 6-6: Rating your food

Several selections are around the house, but the leftover barbecue looks the best. I served myself barbecue, coleslaw, beans, buttered roll, diet soda and a brownie. What I do is taste and rate each food item on the plate. I personally would rate the pork and buttered roll and brownie the highest; coleslaw and beans are least on the list. The brownie (a rich one with pecans) is as high on my list as the juiciest pieces of pork and roll, but I want to save room in my stomach and eat it, too. By the way, sometimes I want a sweet at the end of a meal, but sometimes I do not.

Rating foods will come naturally to you. You have always rated the foods on your plate; however, in the past you ate your least liked foods first and saved the best until the end. Now you will have to reverse that old habit. You will now want to eat your favorite foods first, except for dessert (unless that is what you want). Why? Because you cannot be certain as to when you are going to be full, and once you feel the full feeling, leaving the least-favorite foods on your plate will be easier than leaving the favorite.

I even rate bites inside each category. For example, I searched around in the pork for the juiciest pieces. Since I was approaching full by the time I got to the brownie, I ate the bites that had the most pecans in them. I left some of every food category on my plate, but the juiciest, best morsels were in my stomach. My plate looked as if it had been dissected! And what was left was not appealing. Skinny people eat this way. You will lose weight immediately using these directions. Once you have rated foods for several months, your memory will take over so that you do not have to literally rate every meal.

Leftovers

Somehow the generation that went through the Great Depression birthed a new man-made rule. On top of that, they told the world that it was God's rule. I am referring to the "It is a sin to leave food on your plate while all the children are starving in other parts of the world" rule. In other words, the food is what you obey and bow down to, even if your body has told you, "Enough!" The food has higher value than your own body, and you must obey even though it is literally killing you!

Well, that is certainly not God's line of authority. Food was made
to be a tool to serve mankind, not man to be the slave of food. If it
rots or is wasted—so what! He has more for you.

Look at this passage in Exodus 16:1–5, 20:

The whole Israelite community set out from Elim and came to
the Desert of Sin, which is between Elim and Sinai, on the fifteenth
day of the second month after they had come out of Egypt. In
the desert the whole community grumbled against Moses and
Aaron. The Israelites said to them, "If only we had died by the
LORD's hand in Egypt! There we sat around pots of meat and ate
all the food we wanted, but you have brought us out into this
desert to starve this entire assembly to death."

Then the LORD said to Moses, "I will rain down bread from
heaven for you. The people are to go out each day and gather
enough for that day. In this way I will test them and see whether
they will follow my instructions. On the sixth day they are to
prepare what they bring in, and that is to be twice as much as
they gather on the other days."

However, some of them paid no attention to Moses; they kept
part of it until morning, but it was full of maggots and began to
smell. So Moses was angry with them.

When the Israelites tried to save the food, it turned into maggots.
Several lessons are taught from this passage: obey God, believe that
God will provide for your needs, and trust that God will give you
your daily bread. (And dessert, too!) Do not show a lack of faith in
His completely competent care by being greedy or by getting yourself extra food as if there will be no food for tomorrow. Eat what you
need and then let the rest of the food go. Do not let yourself
or your children be a slave to leftovers. Wrap up leftovers and store
them. Or, if you want to, throw them away. You have God's permission. He cares about you and your happiness—not the food. However, there is nothing righteous about purposely wasting large
amounts of food either. As time goes by, you will learn to cook, take,
or order more appropriate amounts. Your eyes adjust so that less is
put on your plate, and ultimately there will be fewer leftovers.

Eating out

Eating out will be lots of fun! Wait until you know you are good and hungry. Pick the restaurant and choose and order the foods you love the most. Americans are served very large volumes of food; therefore, cut all the food in half. Our experience is that you may feel the full feeling even before you finish the first half. Ask the server for a carryout. Assure the server that the food was wonderful, or he may worry that you were not pleased and therefore worry about the tip. Take the carryout home. If you can, eat it the next time you feel hungry. Do not feel bad about carryouts. These days, it is cool to ask for a carryout even in the finest French restaurants. Many people will split an entree or dessert with someone else, which not only saves money, but also avoids having leftovers when leftovers are inconvenient.

Keep reminding yourself that food is not going to disappear and that your next hunger will come before long.

Your body knows that you are overweight and, therefore, will only ask for a small amount of food. Sometimes, in the course of one day, you will eat all of that during one meal. Sometimes you will eat such small amounts that hunger will occur as many as five times a

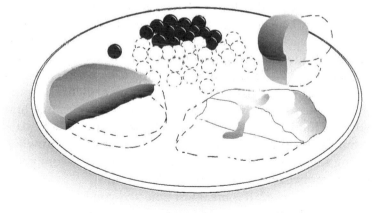

Figure 6-7: Restaurants serve tremendously large portions, so try cutting food portions in half.

day. Basically, the smaller the amount of food you eat at each hunger, the more times your body will ask for food over the course of the day. But if you eat beyond full, you may not feel hunger again until sometime tomorrow. Do not worry about details right now. Just enjoy relearning to eat. Your body loves the decrease in food volumes you have made already! Also do not worry about making a mistake. You can always start over by just waiting for the next hunger. We suggest that you keep a Travel Diary (a sample is provided in Appendix D) to record your journey from Egypt—from the slavery of dieting into the Desert of Testing—a place to learn to trust in God and learn what is in your heart.

How can a family manage?

First of all, your family is going to love this. Regular foods forever! You may worry that if every family member eats on demand, you will become a short-order cook. What's more, you may be concerned that family members might never eat together again. Do not worry; they will!

One fact you need to know to manage this is that you can, quite simply, skip hunger and wait for the next hunger signal. Unlike what the world thinks, this is not painful. The empty sensation will last only ten minutes and will come back again in forty-five minutes to an hour. Your body realizes that you cannot get to food, so it just mobilizes a snack off your hips and feeds your body cells with your stored fat! Knowing this fact, let us look at a few social situations.

Social Situation #1: You are hungry at 5 P.M., but the family usually eats at 6 P.M. Let that first hunger go by, which takes about five to ten minutes. I usually drink a diet drink to help the first hunger go by. The fluid in the stomach seems to help. Now wait to eat with the family whether the hunger symptoms (stomach growling or burning sensation) have come back or not. I will assure you that you are empty enough. Enjoy the guilt-free meal.

Social Situation #2: It is breakfast time and you have always been told that breakfast is the most important meal—that skipping it will make you have cravings and be more out of control and lower your IQ. Wrong. *Another man-made rule!* If you are not hungry—do not eat. You'll do great and your IQ will not drop. (See Appendix B for guidance for the growing child.)

Social Situation #3: What if you are a schoolteacher and you can eat only at 11 A.M. every day—but you are not hungry? If you get hungry between 11 and 3 o'clock, you can wait until the 3 o'clock bell, or you could eliminate or cut back on the volume of breakfast so that you *will* be hungry at 11 A.M. Eventually, you will get the hang of meeting your teaching or work schedule.

Social Situation #4: You ate a big meal during a late afternoon business luncheon with some friends. You are still full. You know that you are not hungry, but it is time to eat with the family. Just sit down with the family and drink your artificially sweetened tea. I bet no one will even notice that you are not eating! You can spend more time enjoying your family.

Social Situation #5: You are in a hurry and you only have ten minutes to eat. The answer is to eat in ten minutes.

In summary, do not panic. You have plenty of stored or emergency meals on your hips or gut. You will get used to smaller amounts of food and this new way to eat (or, in some cases, not eat) while the family is eating. I can still remember when I first started trying God's principles of sacrifice. I remember cooking the food and serving the food and enjoying watching others eat it rather than eating it myself. It was and still is a great feeling. Why, it *is* better to give than it is to receive! God's truths are amazing!

Do not become legalistic about your new rules for eating. There is great flexibility, for the only major rule will be to transfer this heart of love for food over to God. The results will be smaller amounts of food consumed and a smaller you.

What to expect for your first hunger

In summary, start now, not Monday, to wait for stomach hunger. You will feel better than you have in a long time. The body loves it when you do not force food down the esophagus.

Look for a small, empty feeling or growl. Some people have had to wait three hours; some have had to wait a day and a half. The more pounds you have to lose or the bigger the last binge was, the longer the wait for your first hunger. After your first hunger, it may come around one to four times per day, depending on how soon you stop eating or how small each eating occasion is.

If you get a headache, it is probably from the strain of a new focus on resisting the temptation to eat. Just take something for the headache, and pray for strength. The tension will end. Ask God for a clear signal of hunger. Make sure you drink only water or artificially sweetened drinks while waiting. Do not make a habit of chewing sugared gum, hard candy, or your nails or constantly drinking volumes of coffee, diet drinks, or water.

We suggest that you go ahead and eat a small amount of food at the end of thirty-six hours whether you have felt hunger or not, and then start the process over. Hunger should come soon thereafter. If you did not overdo it, it is possible that a headache is a sign of hunger. Keep praying for God to show you. The point is not the legalism of hunger and fullness; the point is to ask God to help you be less greedy for food and to come to Him instead. You *will* get the hang of this.

Once hunger comes, *hallelujah!* Have fun selecting what your heart desires. After all, God programmed your taste buds to like what they like, and He makes no mistakes. Approach the food like a normal eater—someone not greedy or fearful. Start by serving yourself half of what you used to eat or by cutting the food in half. Taste each item. Eat smaller bites and savor each one. Sip your drink between bites to wash the palate off so you can start over and savor the next bite. As you approach full, eat the tastiest morsels first. Leave behind the least-favorite, dry, messy-looking bites. Stop when the little pouch (stomach) feels politely full. Wrap up the leftovers and save them for later or ask for a carryout. Keep telling yourself that you can eat the next time you get hungry. Food is everywhere and, after all, if you are in your thirties, you could have anywhere from 70,000 to 90,000 more eating occasions! Remember, the sooner you stop eating at a meal, the sooner hunger will come back around again.

Last but not least, *thank* God for taking you out of Egypt and the slavery to diets, fat grams and have-to exercise regimens. You will never have to diet *again!* Thank Him for His ingenious food concoctions and creations. What a delight! Food will taste so much better when you are really hungry!

Guess what! We have started thousands of people in the Weigh Down Workshop*, and they all start out searching for this hunger. Much to their surprise and glee, they *find true physiological hunger signals!*

So what should *you* expect in the next few hours? A happy, fulfilled heart and your God-given hunger signal telling you it is now time to eat.

Special situation—What if I cannot find hunger?

Anywhere within one to thirty-six hours, 99 percent of Weigh Down Workshop* starters find hunger—but some of you will not at first. It is OK; do not worry. We have already told you that if you have not found hunger in thirty-six hours, you should go ahead and eat a small meal. Then just try again. It is quite possible that the symptoms or signals of hunger are there, but you do not recognize them as hunger. The range of signals that indicate hunger can be different. However, the bottom line is that any of the symptoms that you would experience are results of a drop in your blood sugar. That drop in blood sugar is normal. The drop in blood sugar signals the brain that your body needs more fuel (or food).

Ultimately, you will know that you are getting to the "E" for your body if you are losing weight.

Look again at the picture of your blood sugar as it relates to the gas gauge on your car (page 43). The person whose blood sugar has dropped enough to give the stomach a growl is on the "E" or is basically empty. You usually would not stop and fill up your car if it has a full tank of gas, so treat your body the same way.

If your body needs fuel (food) by mouth, then your body will ask you to refuel. The need to refuel (this normal drop in the blood sugar) will be sensed by your brain. The brain will send other signals to different parts of your body to make you aware of the need. There is a range of symptoms that you could feel. For example, you could experience weakness, mild shakiness, slight light-headedness, or slight headaches. Some may have a feeling of burning or an empty, hollow feeling up high in the esophagus or below the belt if the stomach pouch has stretched. It is perfectly fine for you to eat when you experience these symptoms because they could be telling you that your blood sugar has dropped. Perhaps you were so busy that you missed the stomach signal. Ultimately, you will know that you are getting to the "E" for your body if you are losing weight.

If your stomach has not burned or growled, and you eat every time you get a headache—and gain weight—you need to keep searching for your *true* physiological hunger signals and treat the headaches with pain relievers.

A second reason some people cannot find hunger is that they are not allowing themselves to get hungry. They wait part of the day for hunger, but finally give in and eat before the stomach signals hunger. Many times when this happens, they eat too much and go past full. If they overeat enough, it could very well take another twenty-four hours to empty out. The next day, they repeat this and never experience true stomach hunger. To remedy this problem, people should keep the amounts they eat small enough so the blood sugar level does not take a whole day to drop down again. More importantly, people should just learn to *wait*. The "Stay Awake" chapter will help you with this. Just add a little more time between each eating occasion. You will eventually work up to waiting for hunger. Do not despair.

Another explanation for an inability to get a hunger signal can be attributed to the amount of weight a person needs to lose to start with. People who are one hundred or more pounds overweight sometimes report going three and four days in the beginning trying to sense hunger. There is a physiological reason that very overweight people might not sense hunger in the early days of this program. The body so desperately wants to shed the excess fat that every time the blood sugar drops, the body will dump fuel from the energy reserves into the bloodstream. The blood sugar goes back up, and the brain does not send any signals or messages to make the stomach growl. Incredibly, as we have said before, the body is getting breakfast from one hip and lunch from the other, so to speak. This confirms how well designed the body is and how desperately it actually desires to burn the stored fuel! Rejoice! This delay will not last; regular hungers will start coming.

The diet industry will tell you that fasting is not good for you and that missing a meal may make it harder to lose weight later, but that is wrong. You will feel better than you have in a long time. Be patient and relax about the amounts of food that you get to eat. Obviously, people who are very large do, in fact, care a great deal for food. Otherwise, they would never have been able to gain so much weight.

So how do you tolerate the periods of time between eating occasions? The answer involves prayer and help from God. A practical thing you can try is to eat one to three small meals over the course of a day. Limit their volume so you can get used to small meals. You can try eating what will fit on a salad plate no more than one to three times per day. Do not cheat. The food should not be hanging off the side of the plate. And do not stack it high either—just small servings on a small plate. Pray that your desire for a lot of food will disappear. Something like this:

Lord, You made my body and set within me the amounts of fuel that are required to live. I pray that You would help me today to be sensitive to those amounts and not to go beyond what is needed. Lord, help me to let go of my focus on food so I will not lust for more than that. Fill my thoughts, instead, with Your love and compassion so I do not feel yearning or greed, but contentment.

You will soon begin to sense the signals of hunger, and then you can switch over to eating only according to hunger and fullness. Make sure you are not "eating" antacids. This will keep the stomach from growling!

If you can tolerate the longer periods of time to just wait for hunger, go ahead. Spend time just bingeing on (reading) the Word of God. You *will* feel full, and your weight loss could be amazingly rapid. This will be covered in more detail in Phase II of this book and in some of the testimonies in Appendix A. You have spent years disregarding your body's signals. You need to see others who feel good from following their bodies' signals. Pray for a focus on God and not on your fears. *You will get there.*

Special situation—My stomach feels as if it burns all the time!

As you begin this new way of eating less food, keep in mind that your body has done its best to adapt and adjust to the extremes of large meals or binges and the starvation or deprivation you have given it through the years. One of the ways the body has adapted is by producing enough stomach acid to accommodate or digest the huge amounts of food you have been eating. The amount of stomach acid that is produced is a "supply and demand" kind of deal. The more that is needed, the more that will be produced. As you need less, the supply will taper off to adjust to the need. Before the Weigh Down Workshop[†], your stomach did not know if it was going to swallow 10,000 calories or just swallow a liquid diet drink because your head or a sheet of paper, not your stomach, decided what and how much to eat.

It will take some time to adjust. For most participants, this is about one to three weeks, but rest assured that hyperacidity will go away.

The hyperacid condition can play a role in after-meal indigestion. Occasionally, you may feel burning right after eating. If you know that you did not overeat, then the burning is just one of the sensations of hyperacidity or too much stomach juices.

If you have overeaten over the years, the sphincter (a circular, muscular ring at the base of the esophagus that keeps food in the stomach) may be weakened. The sphincter's normal position is tightly closed. If it is relaxed or the stomach is overly full, reflux of the acidic food and fluids occurs. The acid then comes in contact

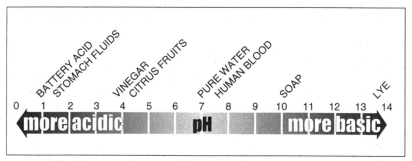

Figure 6-8: Food must become very acidic before it can leave the stomach. Antacids can work against the body's natural digestive process.

with the sensitive lining of the esophagus and causes the burning sensation called heartburn. Avoid lying down after eating if you experience it.

What about antacids? Sometimes, taking a small amount might help, but please do not eat antacids as if they were candy. Antacids reduce the acidity of stomach fluids, making them more basic. Acidity is measured on a pH scale of one to fourteen, with seven being neutral. Acidity increases as the pH number goes down. A fluid with a pH of 4 is ten times more acidic than one with a pH of 5 (see Figure 6-8). Before the food can leave the stomach, the acidity has to increase to 1.5 on the pH scale. That is very acidic. Taking an antacid will delay the moving of the food from the stomach to the small intestine. Be moderate in all things. Let the body adjust, naturally.

Special situation—Effects of illness on hunger

The more you understand about the human body, the more you just have to believe that God is such an incredible genius. One of the systems He created which works in amazing ways is the circulatory system, which includes the heart and blood vessels. Your body can hold only so much blood, so there is a way that your body can direct more or less blood to different parts of the body as needed. For example, if you are studying or taking a test, your body needs a little extra of your blood to supply oxygen and fuel to the brain. The blood vessels in your brain dilate or get bigger, and some of the rest of the blood vessels in your body constrict or get smaller. This allows the blood to go to the area with the greatest need. When you exercise, the blood goes to your muscles. When you eat, it goes to your gut to digest the food. That is why you get sleepy after eating—there is not as much blood in your brain! The more you eat, the sleepier you get.

When you become sick or injured, the blood will go to the area affected by the attacking virus or injury. That is why wounds swell and become red. As a result of the body's attempts to send blood to the sick area, the body will not send a lot of blood to your gut. Likewise, your body balances competing needs for energy. Fighting a virus expends energy, as does digesting food. Therefore, your body will not call for very much food during the time of illness or injury.

It does not want to take the precious blood or energy from the area that needs it the most. So naturally, you can expect that you will not be as hungry as you normally are. By understanding that, you can relax and not try to "feed" the fever, illness, or injury. Mothers and grandmothers want you to eat when you are sick; however, you need to follow the body's cues. Just pay attention to your fluid intake (thirst), and you will heal faster. Feeding the body when it is not asking to be fed is generally not good. However, for some rare conditions, eating despite lack of hunger may be indicated. For example, the chemicals administered during certain cancer treatments may throw the body off balance. Check with your physician and dietitian.

Special situation—Taking medications

Very few medications make a significant impact on appetite and digestion. Even the strongly accused steroid or cortisone is not enough to keep you from being able to lose weight on this program. True physiological hunger can still be sensed and distinguished from side effects of medications. Usually, telling people "This might make your appetite go up or make you gain weight" gives them an open invitation to binge. What would have been a justifiable half-pound weight gain because of the medication becomes a fifteen-pound weight gain because of an inordinate focus on the food, with the blame going to the medication.

In addition, some people use food as a source of comfort during the frustrating time of illness. When the principles of hunger and fullness are applied, then the excuses and overeating will end.

If the medication needs to be taken with food, then there are a couple of things you can do. Wait and take the medication when you become hungry, or if it is a timed medication that has to be taken at 10 A.M., then just have one to three crackers with it. The typical need for food with a pill is to help alleviate the possibility of some irritation to the lining of the stomach. A small amount of food will usually do; you do not need a banquet. Check with your physician.

Special situation—Hypoglycemics and diabetics

All diabetics who decide to apply Weigh Down[1] principles to their eating should consult their physicians. The most common form of diabetes found today is adult-onset diabetes, usually the direct result of overeating. In this condition, the body is overburdened by the ingestion of too much food. The pancreas is simply unable to produce enough insulin to handle the excess food. Insulin acts as a "gatekeeper" to the cells; it enables food to enter the cells. When too little insulin is produced to accommodate this process, food remains in the bloodstream in the form of glucose (blood sugar, or blood food), and the result is an elevated blood sugar level. And when it is elevated, it can spill over into the urine—something that only happens when the kidneys are stressed.

It follows that simply reducing the intake of food will help get the insulin-to-food intake ratio closer. The key is to eat only the amount the body is calling for and not to eat too much food before the bloodstream is ready for more! A few good rules of thumb for adult-onset diabetics just starting out in this program are:

1. Do not start off by fasting.
2. Begin each day following the customary eating pattern recommended by your doctor. Then, in the late afternoon or evening, after you know you have stabilized your blood sugar, start looking for hunger. Fight *desire eating* in the evening hours, the time when most overeating occurs. It will not hurt you at all to cut back; it will help you. Obviously, as you decrease your food intake, you must decrease your insulin intake proportionally. See your doctor.
3. Enjoy a variety of foods at all eating occasions. You can include a small amount of sweets (five or ten M&Ms) if you desire. Small amounts of sweets eaten during or immediately after a meal are tolerated by most adult-onset diabetics.

Juvenile-onset diabetics can also adopt the Weigh Down Workshop[†] approach and do well. All diabetics must make sure that they stay under their physician's care.

Hypoglycemics respond wonderfully to this way of eating. We counsel them to respond to hunger and fullness with sensitivity. By

Testimony from a Juvenile-Onset Diabetic

Through God's Grace the Workshop has been responsible for many changes in my life. Most important is my spiritual growth. I find myself reading God's Word more now than ever. I pray and seek His will much more often. Not only do I pray and seek His will but I also ask for His help with controlling my hunger feelings as well as the problems in my everyday life. Even if I had not lost a single ounce while in Weigh Down, this growth in my spiritual life has been worth any price paid for the program. Please don't misunderstand my thoughts, all of us as Christians know that God's grace and our salvation is a free gift and can't be purchased at any price.

The physical changes that have taken place are to me simply icing on the cake compared to the spiritual growth I have experienced. Now let me tell you a little bit about that icing.

I have been a Class 1, totally insulin dependent, two-shot-a-day diabetic for the past 33 years, since I was nine years old. As a general rule my diabetes has been pretty well under control, but my weight over the past few years has been ever so slowly increasing. A few pounds a year, nothing to worry about, right? *Wrong!*

In January of 1993, my doctor told me I needed to lose about 30 pounds. Well, after a couple of attempts to diet I had only gained four pounds. Then I began to notice that some good friends at my church, Cheryl and Troy, were starting to disappear before my very eyes, weight-wise that is. When I asked them how they were able to lose their weight, they told me all about the Weigh Down program. Troy told me that he would be starting a class. Seeing such good results, I decided to sign up. After sharing a good final meal with my family, I started my first class of Weigh Down, and my journey through the wilderness toward the "Promised Land" began.

I caution anyone who is a diabetic like me or people who have physical problems to seek the advice of their doctor before starting this program. They should also get on their knees and seek God's advice before they start. Personally, I had very good results with the program, and except for some adjustments in my insulin injections, I had no problems adjusting to the new eating habits. But as we all know, everyone is different.

What the Lord did for me that first night and has continued to do for me many times since is something I will never forget. I had made a vow to wait for true stomach hunger before I ate. I had even made it through the 10 P.M. late night snack time without eating. Anyway, at about 2:30 in the morning I woke from a deep sleep. I must have been dreaming of a peanut butter and jelly sandwich. When I woke, the first thing I thought of was the food in the refrigerator. Then I thought of what Gwen had told us about asking the Lord for help when we had desire eating. I was not hungry, so instead of going to the refrigerator, I knelt by my bed and prayed. I asked the Lord to fill me with His spirit and to take away the hunger feeling I had.

The false hunger feeling left immediately. I went back to sleep and didn't eat a bite for hours. Praise God, what a filling of His Spirit can do! Ever since that first night, if a temptation creeps into my mind to eat when I am not really hungry, I simply ask God to fill me with His Spirit. Believe me, it works.

To make a long story a little shorter, in five months I was able to lose 44 pounds. Years later, I haven't gained or lost a single pound. My doctor was impressed, to say the least. I am now able to take half the insulin that I used to take and feel great (plus save money). No longer do I have heartburn and indigestion every day as I used to. The fact is I never get it anymore, which is good because I never did like antacids anyway. I sleep better and have a lot more energy. One thing I can do now that I once could not is bend over, tie my shoes, and talk at the same time. I don't remember all of the measurements that I took of myself, but somewhere I have managed to misplace 10½ inches from my abdomen and 4½ inches from my waist measurements.

There are many more good things I could tell you, but I feel that I must tell you some of the things that are going to regrettably happen to you if you are successful in losing weight. First you will have people asking if you have been sick. Then you are probably going to hurt your mother's feelings because you didn't eat double helpings of her Sunday dinner that she worked so hard to prepare. Sorry, this one really hurts: you are going to have to go and buy some new clothes because the old ones just don't seem to fit anymore!

Wayne R. Russell, Mississippi

doing that, they will no longer go past hunger and risk the severe drops in sugar levels that they experienced in the past. Blood sugar levels become regulated and there are no more extremes.

Special situation—Metabolism

Some people have been told that if they have been on a lot of diets— diet pills or liquid fasts—their metabolism may be altered and their bodies will be resistant to losing weight. To the contrary, we have seen that the minute people start eating less food, they lose weight.

Think about it—how could food companies put calorie counts on the side of a package if everyone had a skewed metabolism? Metabolism refers to the amount of energy (calories) your body traps from food. Everyone traps 80 calories from a slice of bread—even though some of you feel like you will trap 160 calories just by smelling it, while your thin friends can eat five slices of bread and trap only ten calories! Our metabolisms are fine (although, in some very rare cases, people may have disorders such as hypothyroidism). People need different amounts of food to keep their bodies alive, but this is actually related to how much muscle mass they have. Muscle is the most metabolically active tissue. In other words, it takes more calories to keep a muscle cell active than a brain cell. Your body will accurately call for the needed amounts of oxygen and calories. My body has very little muscle mass and what little I have is not exercised much, so I need less food than most adults I know. I am content with a small amount of food.

Special situation—Irregularity

Expect less frequent bowel movements. Do not confuse that with constipation. As your volume of food goes down, so will the excretion level. It is normal to go to the bathroom less frequently. Bran cereals in small amounts with plenty of fluids help alleviate true constipation (hard, dry stools). Contrary to what you have heard, roughage from vegetables has not proven to help with constipation and has been known to cause discomfort.

How to Feed the Stomach

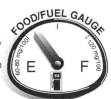

1. Wait anywhere from one to thirty-six hours on your first hunger, and then it will come approximately one to three times a day. Do not fear—you will love the energy you feel from this and the delight from being able to wait.

2. Hunger is a polite burning sensation, the feeling of a knot inside your stomach. If you have to bypass hunger due to work or social conflicts, the sensation will come back around in forty-five minutes. While it is normal to skip hunger once in a while, do not make it a habit. If you haven't felt hunger within thirty-six hours, eat a small meal and wait for hunger again. You should feel it soon. After your first attempt, do not keep waiting thirty-six hours. Continue to decrease your food daily until you feel stomach hunger. Do not be legalistic. We are working on reducing food intakes to normal amounts for your body.

3. Family meal time. If you are hungry before dinner, just bypass hunger. If you are full at normal mealtime because of an irregular eating schedule or because you tasted all your cooking—several times—then just drink a glass of non-caloric tea and talk to the family.

4. Drink non-caloric beverages to help the sugar levels drop normally so that you can get the hunger signal. Continual intake of sugar through drinks prevents you from sensing hunger.

5. Sip your drink between bites. Stop eating when you are satisfied.

6. Rate foods. Decide which foods you like best and eat those first, saving the least favorite until the end. Generally, leave desserts until last.

7. Wrap up the leftovers. You can have them the next time you are hungry.

8. Use carryouts when eating out. Restaurants serve such large portions. Some foods, especially pastas, taste better the next day. Some just turn green in the fridge, and then you can easily throw them away!

9. Do not serve yourself a five-course meal just because a medication must be taken with food. Food needed with pills can be small amounts like one to three crackers. You do not need a banquet unless the physician orders that.

10. In the Weigh Down Workshop[†] expect your food consumption to decrease from 1/2 to 2/3 of what you were eating as an overeater. As you progress, you may expect your desire eating, or desire for food, to decrease over time.

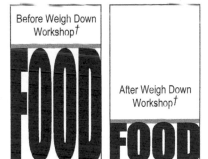

Before Weigh Down Workshop[†]

After Weigh Down Workshop[†]

PHOTOCOPY AND CARRY THIS WITH YOU AS A REMINDER

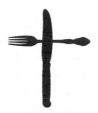

HELP! I FEEL
HUNGRY ALL THE TIME

Once you begin to wait for true physiological hunger, you discover that there is another feeling of hunger. It is your own "I'm not hungry, but I want it anyway" will. We will call this *desire eating*, or head hunger. To help you understand this idea, imagine a headstrong two-year-old child, prone to temper tantrums, who sees a toy, desires it, beats his hands on the floor to speed up the service, grabs the toy, and hoards it.

The emptier our souls are, the stronger the *desire eating* is. This *desire eating* has grown so over the years that it might even have turned into a monster. It is ravenous, headstrong, willful and self-loving. It feels like a magnetic force to the refrigerator that controls you rather than your controlling it.

We think we love food, we love the taste, we love the feeling of control. We love a secret rendezvous with food. We love to put our children to bed and have no one present to tell us what to do or to judge us. We love to fulfill the *desire eating* binge at 10 P.M. with foods we have been secretly dreaming of all day long.

Why do we do this? We love the comfortable *feeling* of eating as much as we want. In fact, we love that *desire eating* so much that we have ignored the physical pain of overeating, such as the over-stretched stomach pouch, the pain of the dumping syndrome of diarrhea, or the pain of gastric reflux in the esophagus. We have also ignored the chronic pain of the overweight condition—clothes too tight, joints that hurt, and fatigue. However, at the end of the binge we feel awful about ourselves, and our guilt leads to a feeling of depression.

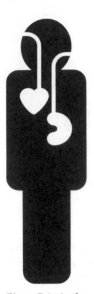

When we binge or graze without having any physiological hunger, we are looking for a feeling. *Looking for a feeling* is not wrong. God is the Creator of you and the Creator of feelings; therefore, it is OK to look for a feeling. However, if you go to the physical world or anything in or on this world to get the *feeling* of comfort, fulfillment, love or control, you may get it only *temporarily*. But it will disappear and leave you with an even larger gnawing, longing, wanton need than you had before.

The world cannot satisfy. This is true if you go after the intoxicated feeling, the antidepressant feeling, the feeling of sexual lust, the tobacco feeling, the love of money feeling, or the love of the praise of people feeling. After you taste the world and its pleasures, you are empty and you are left in need *again*. You become even more out of control and desperate.

Figure 7-1: As the heart fills up with love from God, the desire to "feed" the soul with physical food disappears.

But when you feed your longing soul with a search for God, His will, and His personality; and when you experiment with talking to Him, doing things His way, getting your prayers answered because you did things His way, trusting Him, and liking Him; then you finally fall in love with Him. Love for God fills your heart, and the old empty feeling leaves *permanently*.

You start to feel full, fulfilled, not so "hungry" anymore. Panic disorders disappear and anger dissipates. Your "making it happen" goals are not needed as you simply look to God to make it happen. He answers prayers.

What transpires in this transfer is that the ravenous *desire eating* starts to fade and the true stomach hunger starts to emerge. True stomach hunger is much easier to find as this "desire to just feed yourself" fades.

One of the most practical things you can do with the *desire eating* feeling is to walk away from it and into a private room to talk to God. (Of course, you can talk to Him in your car or in a room full of people—the location does not stop communication.) I have taught many people just to open up the Word and start reading wherever their eyes fall. God can coordinate personal communication with us. One person took my advice, and she just cried out to God and asked if He even cared. She opened her Bible, and her eyes fell to this passage from Psalm 81:4–10:

> . . . this is a decree for Israel,
>   an ordinance of the God of Jacob.
> He established it as a statute for Joseph
>   when he went out against Egypt . . .
> He says, "I removed the burden from their shoulders;
>   their hands were set free from the basket.
> In your distress you called and I rescued you,
>   I answered you out of a thundercloud;
>   I tested you at the waters of Meribah.
> "Hear, O my people, and I will warn you —
>   if you would but listen to me, O Israel!
> You shall have no foreign god among you;
>   you shall not bow down to an alien god.
> I am the LORD your God,
>   who brought you up out of Egypt.
> Open wide your mouth and I will fill it."

"Open wide your mouth and I will fill it," says the Lord! She started crying because God was personally communicating to her. At that moment a relationship started that has grown more and more.

"For God does speak— now one way, now another— though man may not perceive it" (Job 33:14). In my personal life, I cling to my Bible as I used to cling to my chocolate! I keep my eyes open, looking for God's guidance everywhere.

Another practical thing to do with *desire eating* is to talk to the food and tell it that you are not going to answer to *it* anymore. You will not obey it when it calls your name from the kitchen cabinets or refrigerator!

Do not be afraid of running to God. He is your Father! And He has the finest personality. I could not describe to you a richer, more powerful, just, and moral being.

I am really excited for what is ahead for you! One day, after your normal lunch time, you will suddenly realize that you have not even thought about food because your stomach has not signaled you to eat. Congratulations! *Stomach hunger,* rather than *head hunger* (or *desire eating*), is beginning to control your eating! And you will also discover that you are beginning to feel closer to God. The transfer is underway!

It was not so crazy to try to fill up your spiritual void or emptiness with food. You have simply made a mistake: you chose physi-

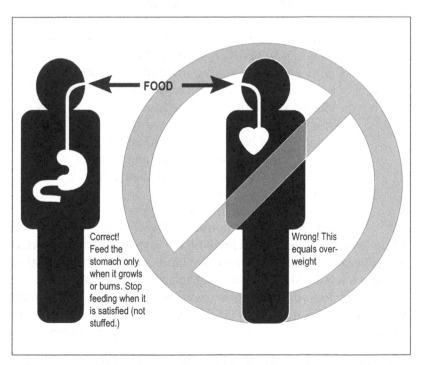

Figure 7-2: *You will become better at distinguishing head hunger from stomach hunger.*

cal, earthly food when what you really needed was spiritual food, a give-and-take relationship with God. Believe me, He will be doing most of the giving and you will be doing most of the taking. "I am the LORD your God, who brought you up out of Egypt. Open wide your mouth and I will fill it."

Open yourself to Him right now, and He will fill your heart. *Desire eating* will soon disappear if you run to the Bible or to prayer every time you feel this urge to eat when the stomach is *not* calling for food.

ISN'T BROCCOLI RIGHTEOUS AND HÄAGEN-DAZS A SIN?

I want you to know that I love God with all my heart and that I have gotten to know Him so much better over the years. I have also read a lot of God's recorded ideas in the Bible. I have observed the world He made and watched His animals eat. I have watched children eat. God's eating plan is plastered everywhere, and we have just missed it. He has put food down on earth for us to enjoy, and He did not accidentally leave the Basic Four food groups out of the Bible. He did not put food down here to torture us.

Also, it is more His idea *not* to worry about what we eat or drink. If God bothers to feed the little birds or if He bothers to clothe the flowers in the field, which live only for a couple of weeks and then are gone, will He not feed and clothe you—a human being, made in His likeness and possessing a life span of eternity? Matthew 6:25 recorded Jesus' words this way: " 'Therefore I tell you, do not worry about your life, what you will eat or drink; or about your body, what you will wear. Is not life more important than food, and the body more important than clothes?'"

So God does not want us to worry excessively about getting

enough food to eat. He does not want us to worry about the food's content, as we learned earlier in Mark 7:14–23.

In this passage, you recall, Jesus declared all foods clean. God gave food rules to the Israelites, but all along He wanted the heart or the core of man's character to be pure and loving and devoted only to Him. He sent Jesus, the exact representation of God's being, the radiance of God's glory (Hebrews 1:3), to show us that God wants us to work on the heart's being pure, rather than work on making the environment pure.

So we can conclude that physical food should not be the focus, but rather spiritual food should be the food for the heart. And we should likewise be praying for our spiritual concerns and spiritually clogged arteries instead of just praying for people with physical ailments.

It turns out that most of us like to be around personalities who love us, who think we are "it" or something special. When we seek to know God, we quickly discover His deep affection for us, how very special we are to Him. It then becomes very easy—and easier as time goes by—to make God the object of our own affection. I am personally crazy about Him; I cannot get Him off my mind. As your heart changes from a love for food to a love for God, you will find another amazing transformation happening. You will not be consumed with food *content*, its nutritional value, or whether it is good or bad for you. The color green will no longer seem virtuous, and your obsessive-compulsive worry of whether something is "organic," "natural," or "chemical-free" will evaporate. A small amount of food will do nicely. And best of all, your hunger is satisfied—*all* of your hunger.

The scientific explanation

After earning an undergraduate degree in dietetics and a master's degree in nutrition science, I came to the exact opposite conclusion of what was taught in my university classes. I concluded that you do not have to worry about what you eat if you use your God-given cues to guide you. The body does 99 percent of the worrying (work) for you. This understanding probably resulted from my confidence in a very coordinated, ingenious Heavenly Father.

Dietetics is mostly biochemistry, since everything you eat is a chemical and every cell in your body and your bloodstream is just chemicals—primarily carbon, hydrogen, oxygen, and nitrogen. Nutrition and dietetics are the study of the chemicals that your body manufactures for you. For example, you do not have to eat brain cells to have brain cells! Your body manufactures them. (Too bad— I could use some more!)

It is interesting to note that health food stores will sell you food chemicals that your body manufactures, such as lecithin. You do not need to eat lecithin—it is produced by your liver!

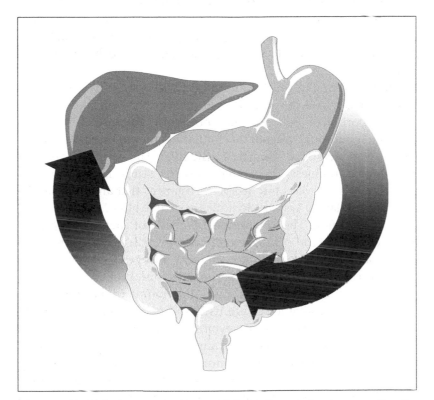

Figure 8-1: Food is broken apart in the stomach, broken down further to very small units in the small intestine, taken to the liver to be converted to usable substances, and then sent to the bloodstream via the hepatic vein to the heart.

Dietetics is also the study of the consumption and digestion of chemicals the body does not manufacture and, therefore, needs to receive by mouth. What I learned from the study of biochemistry is that our bodies are wonderfully made and that most of their workings remain beyond the reach of our intellect. We do know much of what our body systems do, but we still know only a fraction of how they do it or what makes them do it. How we, from just two cells, can reproduce another human being's body to have all the bodily functions and incredible ability to live is so amazing. The study of just the two functions of digestion and absorption is mind-boggling! Spending hours with the books brought me to one major conclusion: there is a Creator who is more intelligent than I. Even if we could finally fathom all systems of the human body, we could not reproduce another human being. Some people are amazed at twins. I am amazed that God has managed to create so much variety in all of us.

From studying chemistry and biochemistry, we can see that our bodies take what we eat and break it down to tiny molecules or units. A portion of these now tiny food units can cross the intestinal wall and go through a separate circulating system that leads breakfast, lunch and supper directly to the liver. The liver is a large (silent, thank goodness) organ that converts Fritos, M&Ms, Doritos and dip, and Twinkies into usable substances that are sent into the regular circulatory system. So how are people alive?

Good question. The food you eat is made of chemicals—primarily molecules of carbohydrates, fats, and proteins—which are made up of carbons, hydrogens, oxygen, and nitrogen (see Figure 8-2). After you swallow the food, it is shredded and broken apart by the acid in the stomach. It moves in small amounts to the small intestine, where digestive juices are used to break down the carbohydrates, fats, and proteins into even smaller units. These units are moved across the intestinal walls and to the liver—a process taking anywhere from five to twenty minutes. Dietary fats (also called triglycerides) do not go directly to the liver. After crossing the intestinal wall, they take a longer trip, slowly moving between the body's cells in a space called the lymphatic system. Triglycerides will drip into the regular bloodstream through the various ducts and then finally circulate to the liver. This route can take up to thirteen hours. The slow entry keeps the blood sugar stabilized. If you eat a meal that is primarily carbohydrates, you will be hungry sooner. If you add fats, it will help you go longer before you feel hungry again.

The liver is amazingly designed to take the broken-down food units—proteins, carbohydrates, and fats—and turn the largest per-

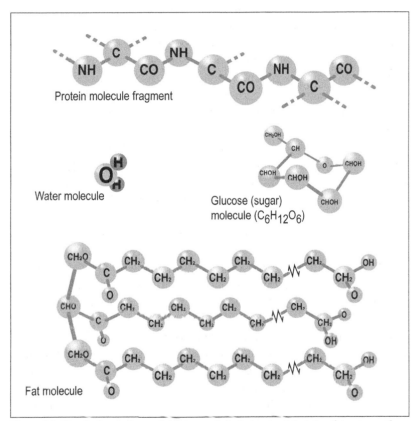

Figure 8-2: Your body can turn a fat into a carbohydrate, a protein into a fat, or any other combination of the three. In other words, you can take a carbohydrate, fat, or protein, and change one into the other. Most of what you eat is broken into those small units and turned into glucose molecules to feed each cell. These chemical reactions take place in the liver. Notice the carbon (C), hydrogen (H), oxygen (O), and sometimes nitrogen (N) in all these structures. If you overeat a carbohydrate, fat, or protein, it is turned into a fat and shipped to your body's favorite storage locations—the gut and the hips.

centage of these into glucose (the body's fuel or energy source). So you are *not* exactly what you eat. The liver takes what you have eaten and, via chemical reaction, reforms the units into the substances the human body needs. These newly-made substances are moved into the hepatic vein that goes to the heart. Once they reach the heart, they enter the main circulatory system and are pumped all over the body, giving each cell what it needs.

All foods are composed of just water, proteins, carbohydrates, fats, and trace (tiny) amounts of vitamins and minerals. Proteins, carbohydrates (CHO), and fats are made up of carbon, hydrogen, and oxygen. Proteins add nitrogen to their chemical structures.

These are organic molecules; *organic* means that the molecule contains carbon. You do not have to go to the health food store for good organic foods. They are displayed at every grocery store and corner market.

If organic means *chemical-free* to you, think again. All foods are chemicals. God made your body (without your having to worry about it!) to detect and rid itself of harmful chemicals that are part of the normal dietary process. Let us say your child just accidentally ate a serving of mud or some dirt. His stomach would be the first place that could detect harmful bacteria or chemicals. The stomach may throw it back up and out of the body. Most harmful bacteria would be destroyed in the very acidic (pH 1.5) stomach fluids. If harmful substances get past the stomach and into the intestines, then the body might trigger diarrhea (increased peristalsis) to rid the body of them. If they make their way through the walls of the small intestine (it is very difficult for most foreign objects or harmful substances to make it past this barrier) and then to the liver, the liver will trap them, break them apart, and render them unavailable and incapable of harming your child or his liver.

Just think—your child might have been watching a movie while all this was going on, oblivious to this chemical factory inside him. The point is this: "organic foods" and grocery store foods are *both* organic in that they contain carbon (which, as we said earlier, means they are organic). No matter how someone grows them, they both will have picked up the normal sprinkling of harmful substances. So if you like foods advertised as being "organic," fine. Just do not count on their being better for you . . . just more expensive.

Another point: you do not have to count exchanges or food groups to have a balanced meal. For the most part, all the food groups contain the six basic nutrients.

For example, when you eat a piece of bread, you think you are eating just a carbohydrate. No, it is largely a carbohydrate, but it also contains proteins, fats, water (H_2O), vitamins, and minerals.

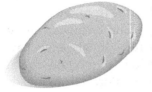

What about a potato? It is made of carbohydrates, a trace of proteins and fat, vitamins, minerals, and water.

What about meat? It is proteins, fat and a trace of carbohydrates, vitamins, minerals, and water.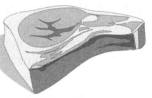

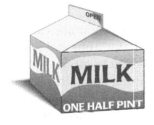

What about milk? Well, it is proteins, carbohydrates, fats, vitamins, minerals, and water, too.

What about chocolate, cookies, cake, or candy?
They, too, are fats, proteins, carbohydrates, a trace of vitamins, minerals, and water.

Simple carbohydrates are made of short chains of glucose (basically $C_6H_{12}O_6$). Breads are made of long chains of glucose. Fructose (another arrangement of $C_6H_{12}O_6$) is a simple carbohydrate that God made to fit exactly in the taste bud, which in turn stimulates a nerve ending to send a signal that the brain interprets as "delightfully sweet." If you were to examine the bloodstream, you would not be able to tell if you had eaten long chains or short chains. Glucose is the sugar form that each of your cells uses for energy. We do not have to eat it—the foods we eat are turned into glucose. Likewise,

your body does not know if it ate honey, unrefined sugar from the
sugar cane plant, refined table sugar, or bread because all the units
are converted to glucose in the liver and then dumped into the bloodstream to be used by the body cells. Being overanxious about the
source of sugar is part of the bondage of food.

Table sugar comes from the sugarcane plant and is extracted in
the form of molasses. Molasses can crystallize, and this is what we
call dark brown sugar. If the syrup is washed off the crystals, you
will have light brown or table sugar, depending on the level of wash-
ing. If table sugar is crushed into smaller pieces, it is then called
powdered sugar. All of these are wonderful gifts from the Father.

While we are talking about carbohydrates and breads, I want to
point out that it is sad to see that so many professional dieters have
gone against the body's need for bread. Much of the non-dieting
Third World countries eat 80 percent of their calories from breads.
Jesus said, "I am the bread of life." That had meaning in Jesus' day
and has meaning to most of the world today. Bread was and still is
the staple. Our point is to not be afraid of reintroducing plenty of
bread. You are going to feel so great when you let yourself go back
to what your body calls for.

All foods have varying combinations of these six units: carbon,
hydrogen, nitrogen, vitamins, minerals and water. Your main need
is for energy or fuel to run the body. We have made eating—something intended to be enjoyable—into something complicated and
burdensome. The food industry has picked up on our fears and has
capitalized on them. If the heart associations have alerted you to be
careful of too much whole milk due to heart disease, then the dairy
associations alert you to be sure to drink milk because of its possible
association with preventing osteoporosis. The chicken industry has
soared while the poor beef industry continues to struggle. I personally love red meat. I enjoy all foods in moderation. I believe this
moderation does not shorten our lives. Ironically, I know the world
tells me I should be dying from eating beef and putting *real* cream in
my coffee, but I am *a-l-i-v-e!* In turn, some nutritionally obsessed
people who shop in or operate health food stores look like they are
dying! Why? It seems to me the more we try to monitor our health,
the unhealthier we get. Let go and listen to what the body calls for.

All animals use this same system for eating. Sensitivity to volume is the dietary habit of most ninety-year-olds. You may know some over-weight sixty-year-olds. But how many overweight ninety-year-olds do you know?

Some of the foods you eat are already in the form that your body calls for. The body just needs to break them down to smaller units. Some of what you eat, such as whole wheat fiber and celery fiber, never even get past the small intestine cell wall and so are excreted in feces.

Other nutrients you need, such as vitamins and minerals, are wide-spread in various foods and are needed only in tiny, tiny amounts. I have worked in the health department in a state which statistics say is one of the poorest in the United States, and I rarely ever docu-mented malnutrition (vitamin deficiency), except in a rare case of parental negligence in feeding a child. But I did, however, docu-ment and chart obesity daily.

My belief is that the lack of a nutrient is highly overemphasized. Some of the most clearly documented cases of true malnutrition (scurvy, beriberi or pellagra) occur when people cannot make the selection for themselves because a variety is unavailable. An example of this occurred years ago when sailors spent months on the sea in non-motorized ships. Early sailing ships were stocked with all the foods available, but as months went by, the variety of food ran out, leaving salt pork and biscuits for breakfast, biscuits for lunch, bis-cuits for supper, and biscuits for the bedtime snack. As a result, the mariners got sick from a lack of variety, usually vitamin C deficiency (scurvy).

It does not take a genius to figure out that this was not a typical eating situation. Everyone knows that only those sailors, wartime prisoners, or neglected children would have to eat the same thing over and over. You cannot force free-to-eat-anything populations into monotonous diets because the body will cue them to desire and consume a variety of foods. The poor sailors were sick of bis-cuits, and anything but biscuits was what they were craving. When the mariners reached shore and resumed eating regular foods, they recovered if caught in time. The British Royal Navy eventually learned to supply a variety of food and, to prevent scurvy, to have plenty of limes on board (thus giving their sailors the nickname "Limeys").

We propose to you that we are *not* what we eat, but that health is adversely affected when we deny the body the kinds and amounts of food it *wants*. The human body, over time, wants a variety of foods.

Another point: species are programmed by God to crave specifically the foods *their* digestive systems were designed for—and we are not what we eat! God has programmed cows to want grass. Does this mean cows turn into grass? No! They not only remain cows, they also produce more cows and produce calcium-rich milk. Do baby whales eat plankton and turn into plankton? Of course not! They turn into giant whales, make more whales, and the mother whales produce milk. Cardinals are programmed to eat sunflower seeds, but they turn into cardinals. Robins eat worms; mockingbirds eat grasshoppers, and they all live to sing about it.

Cats are not really picky eaters. They just need variety and will refuse food when it becomes monotonous—it's biological feedback. Feeding your pets food scraps from the table is perfect variety and could even be considered Biblical (" '. . . even the dogs eat the crumbs that fall from their masters' table' " Matthew 15:27).

We need to reexamine old wives' tales and new man-made scientific rules. For example, as we discussed, we tell our children that if they do not eat breakfast, their IQ will drop (never mind that they ate two bowls of cereal before bed and they are simply *not* hungry). The irony is that overeating makes you sleepy, and that is when intellectual response rates really drop!

"If you don't eat carrots, you will have night blindness. If you don't drink orange juice every morning, you will die!" I got my nerve up to challenge this one eighteen years ago, and I am still alive! Vitamin C is found all through the pantry and refrigerator, and it is even in your french fries and ketchup! God designed nutrients to be widespread in foods so that you do not have to worry. Occasionally, I drink orange juice now.

Why do we live in dread that we or our children are going to miss a trace mineral or miss out on the latest anticancer, longevity cureall? We desperately look for life in all the wrong places and seem convinced that when the Bible was written, God knew nothing about cholesterol, which man discovered in the twentieth century. We think God could not have meant 1 Timothy 4:1–5 to be useful for the junk eaters of today. "The Spirit clearly says that in later times some will abandon the faith and follow deceiving spirits and things taught by demons. Such teachings come through hypocritical liars, whose consciences have been seared as with a hot iron. They forbid people to marry and order them to abstain from certain foods, which God created to be received with thanksgiving by those who believe and who know the truth. For everything God created is good, and nothing is to be rejected if it is received with thanksgiving, because it is consecrated by the word of God and prayer."

We think, "They didn't have fat and processed foods back then. The Bible must be obsolete." But think again. Take a look at Leviticus 2:4–6, 11–13 and the offerings that were eaten way back in time and ordained by God:

" 'If you bring a grain offering baked in an oven, it is to consist of fine flour: cakes made without yeast and mixed with oil, or wafers made without yeast and spread with oil. If your grain offering is prepared on a griddle, it is to be made of fine flour mixed with oil, and without yeast. Crumble it and pour oil on it; it is a grain offering . . . .

" 'Every grain offering you bring to the LORD must be made without yeast, for you are not to burn any yeast or honey in an offering made to the LORD by fire. You may bring them to the LORD as an offering of the firstfruits, but they are not to be offered on the altar as a pleasing aroma. Season all your grain offerings with salt. Do not leave the salt of the covenant of your God out of your grain offerings; add salt to all your offerings.' "

Processed fine flour, spread with oil and salt added—my, that grain offering is very similar to our present-day Frito!

There is nothing new under the sun. John the Baptist ate locusts and honey, and he lived in the desert that way for months. This menu has virtually nothing of the Basic Four food groups or the new food pyramid groups taught today. All this is to say that you are more free with food than you might think.

Fats are not evil. God made fats to "house" the flavor of foods. When you breathe, the fat molecules are picked up by the olfactory cells in your nose. Aroma! That is why you sauté bell peppers and onions in fat. The flavor is trapped into the fat molecules, and you then take the fat mixture and transfer the flavor into your spaghetti or whatever. That is why you smell the bacon cooking, but not the oatmeal—unless you put butter, a fat, in the oatmeal, of course. Fats make the food more palatable and easier to swallow.

By the way . . . I put real butter and sugar in my oatmeal, and I eat butter, salt, and pepper in my grits! Yum!

Now, why would God put fats down on earth to torture us? Why would He ask for the fat portions to be saved for Him as a *pleasant aroma* if it was not something inherently desirable? Look at this verse: "From what he offers he is to make this offering to the LORD by fire: all the fat that covers the inner parts or is connected to them, both kidneys with the fat on them near the loins, and the covering of the liver, which he will remove with the kidneys. The priest shall burn them on the altar as food, an offering made by fire, a pleasing aroma. All the fat is the LORD's" (Leviticus 3:14–16).

Fats are used for many bodily functions and for the health of your hair. Yes, too much fat is bad for you; likewise, too many carrots at one sitting will kill you because vitamin A is toxic in large quantities. But moderation without overindulgence allows us to enjoy *all* food categories, including fats and sweets. I eat them daily.

I do not take vitamin pills, my grandparents did not take them, and my great-grandparents did not, either. If you are looking for good health, then know that the single most related factor to disease and even early death is overeating. Overeating brings added stress and burdens to every organ and system in our body. Our joints hurt, and our stomach hurts (reflux esophagitis, heartburn, diarrhea, hiatal hernias, diverticulitis, etc.). Our blood pressure is higher, and our risk of cancer and heart disease is greater, not to mention the mental and emotional state it puts us in. If you have overeaten, your body does not readily need the excess food. Too much food, even if it is a virtuous salad, has to be taken to the liver, turned into a fat, and shipped to our storage tanks, the hips and gut. No food is virtuous when you overeat, but all foods are "clean" in moderation.

Eating only *when* your body calls for food is what you can depend on to moderate the amount you eat daily. Eating *what* your body asks for will ensure a balance of food. When you have had too much of one category of food, you will naturally desire to eat from another category.

Biological feedback

The Weigh Down Workshop[t] techniques of food consumption involve a threefold learning process. First, you understand hunger.

Second, you recognize fullness and begin to stop at that point.

Third, you develop this ability to sense what your body is really calling for.

To begin developing this ability to sense what your body is calling for, ask yourself, "What do I really want to eat?" Thin eaters try to get what they want, within reason. Some of you have no idea. This response is not unusual at first.

Realize that you may have been dieting for years—perhaps even back to your childhood. Think about it. As a child, you ate what your mother cooked for you. Then you went to school and ate what the cooks prepared. As you got older, you started dieting and ate what the latest piece of paper told you to eat.

Have you ever in your entire life picked what you wanted to eat? Well, no wonder you do not know how to do it! Let me help *you* decide. Just ask yourself, "What really, really sounds good right now?" OK, so you cannot believe that you really want a grilled cheese sandwich, and it is only 8:30 in the morning. Do not worry about it. If that is what you really want, get it, enjoy it, and feel no guilt. Pay attention, however. Your body may only want *half* of a sandwich. Remember that it is the tendency of every new Weigh Down Workshop[t] participant to gravitate toward foods and food categories that they have deprived themselves of for years. Again, what foods do the diets deny you the most? Sweets and fats, right? So do not be afraid if that is the category you want right now. Fats are the nutrients needed for the integrity of your cells and mucosal lining and the health of your hair, etc. You may be needing fats. Let yourself have those foods so that you will not feel deprived. Soon you will want a wider variety.

But what if I know I am hungry and nothing sounds good or if I still cannot figure out what to eat? If nothing "sounds" good, then you could wait a little longer until something does sound good. You might *not* really be that hungry right now. Or, you can try to narrow down the field a little. Ask yourself about some general categories at first. "Do I want something hot or cold? Do I want something salty or sweet? Do I want something crunchy or creamy?" These questions will put you in the general ballpark of some of the food categories to choose from. Some days your cravings will be very specific. For example, a hamburger sure sounds good right now! Within reason, be obedient to what your body is calling for.

Say, for instance, that I have narrowed it down to lasagna. I go to the kitchen, but the lasagna is in the freezer and it would take such a long time to thaw and cook it. So I start looking for something else. At this point, any kind of meat and cheese sounds good, but I'm basically too lazy to fool with it. That is when my eye spots the bag of chips in the pantry. It is not meat, but Weigh Down Workshop[†] did say I could eat anything I wanted, right? So I get the bag of chips and start to eat. For some reason, they do not taste as good as I thought they would, but that is OK. I begin to feel full, so I put back the bag. I know I've had enough because I can feel the volume of food in my stomach and I can tell that my blood sugar has gone back up, but I still "want" something. Do you see what has happened here? I was not obedient to what my body was calling for, so as soon as I finished eating, my body was still crying out for the protein in the meat that I didn't give it! That is why dieting will not work.

Did you notice the point that the chips did not taste as good as usual? That point is important, because it is a clue to you either that you are not really hungry or chips are not the food your body wants right now. Trust your taste buds to guide you in your choices. When you have a plate of food in front of you and you have tasted everything, the items that taste the best are the ones your body needs. The next meal, you desire different foods. Why? Because your body does not want what it had for breakfast. Variety is what your body needs. Actually, variety is what it calls for even within a single meal, much less over a three-day period.

God has made you to prefer something new rather than leftovers for three days in a row. What fun! What a genius He is.

The older I get, the more I believe that you would be hard-pressed to make a big mistake in any selection of foods. Do not be legalistic with choices. Good health is more related to *when* you eat and *how much* you eat than *what* you eat, since most meal selections are so similar in chemical and nutrient content. Keep it simple.

Problem foods and problem times

God made your taste buds. He made you, and He designed you to have likes and dislikes. He knows what your preferences are, so do not be afraid to have favorites, even if they sound as if they are fattening. Do you have a particular favorite food that you seem to have struggled with more than others? What is it? Chocolate, doughnuts, homemade bread? It is not unusual for a particular food to be one that involves years of conflict. Maybe it is a food that you have more passion about, maybe one that you have binged on before. You may even find that you can wait for hunger before eating the chocolate, but then stopping is harder. You want to eat it all!

Let me reassure you that you can indeed rise above *this* passion for food, too. You actually have two choices as to how to approach conquering this "trigger food."

First of all, be reassured that there are no "trigger foods" in the sense that some foods can turn something on inside you and make you lose control. Control is all in the heart of a person, and you *do* have a choice. Do not be afraid.

Let us use chocolate candy bars as an example. One method of reassurance would be to go and buy a bag of candy bars and keep them in your pantry, take some to work with you, and have one every time you are hungry. Your body, as you know, will begin to seek a variety and will put an end to the affection quickly.

The only problem with this approach for some people is that every time they eat one of the candy bars, they eat another . . . then another . . . then another . . . until they have overeaten. It is not that they *cannot* stop, but they *will* not. Believe me, they listen to every lie imaginable to keep eating. "Oh, they will tempt me, so I had better finish them off . . . Everyone else will come in and eat them soon, so I had better have one more before they are all gone." (Like there were no more candy bars at the store!)

This is the route selected by one Weigh Down Workshop[†] participant to conquer her "trigger" or pedestal food. Since she did not trust herself to buy a whole bag of candy bars, she would buy only one at a time. Now, realize that she never denied herself a candy bar any time a candy bar was what she really wanted when she was hungry; she just did not have them sitting around tempting her. She would go to the store, buy her very favorite kind, walk away, and then really enjoy that one candy bar. The next time she wanted a candy bar, she would go buy another and enjoy it, too. After a while, she got up the courage to buy half a dozen. She realized that if she put them in the freezer until she wanted another one, they would keep, and they tasted great. You see, she was beginning to trust. It was not much longer until she could buy a whole bag and not eat them all. Even at work (they had a snack machine), she began to notice that sometimes she just did not want one. Now they are like any other food to her. They are still good, but they just do not have that pedestal beneath them. If she wants one, she will have one; but to be honest, she is not sure when the last time was.

Another helpful tip is to keep a box to put your food in. This is a very elementary idea, but it could be a psychological breakthrough. Get a box and write your name on it. Place one in the pantry, one in the refrigerator, and one in the freezer. This is your property, and no one else in the house can touch the food in your box. Some participants actually open the package of cookies as they unload the newly purchased groceries and put some in a plastic bag for themselves. The family can have the

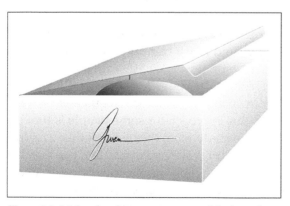

Figure 8-3: Make a box for your own personal food supply.

rest of the package that they place in the pantry. This works well for the person who lives in fear that "If I don't eat it now, it will be gone." For some, it is a lack of trust in God to provide, and for some, this lack of trust stems from growing up in a household where this "eat it or it is gone" phenomenon actually occurred. If fear that the food will be gone is driving you to eat when you are not hungry, then eliminate the source of the fear until you can have the confidence that food really is available abundantly and, more importantly, that God loves to feed you and will never let you starve. Do not be afraid to be caught without food. Take it with you. Keep it in your car, your purse, or your desk at work. Then you can sit back and relax, knowing something good is there if you need it. Food is everywhere!

What about holiday meals? It is Thanksgiving, and you fear you will not get this kind of food again for a whole year! That is simply not true. Who says you cannot buy a turkey and cook it on a different day than Thanksgiving? You can even cook one in July! Or, even better, go to a cafeteria-style restaurant and order some. They serve chicken and dressing or turkey and dressing all year long! What law states you have to eat wedding cake at a reception because you might not get any for a long time? A bakery would be happy to bake a cake for you to take home and eat a slice each time you are hungry! You may become sick of it before it is all gone. What about Aunt Tillie's cherry salad on Christmas Day? Now, you know you get that only once a year. Ask for the recipe. She will probably be flattered, and then you can make it as often as you like. There is no food and no occasion that should cause you to eat outside of the context of hunger! God knows your favorites. Be a little more patient and let Him indulge you with them under His rules: hunger and fullness. And do not be afraid that God's watch is broken or that He has forgotten about you. He is very attentive!

Food allergies

True food allergies should be respected. For instance, if you are allergic to certain seafoods, then by all means, do not eat them. If you know you have a milk sensitivity, listen to your body and limit your milk intake. You will know your own sensitivities, hungers, and nutritional needs. Use common sense. However, there are many more incidents of simple food sensitivities that are not true allergies. You might try tiny portions of these foods and see how your body responds. Let your body tell you if it wants or needs or does *not* want certain foods. Also, since your portions are now so greatly reduced, you may discover that you experience no reaction at all when you eat foods you were formerly sensitive to. It is very hard to truly know whether diarrhea is an allergic reaction from a food or from a virus. It is hard to determine whether a skin rash is from a food or a new laundry detergent. Do not jump to conclusions. Any severe conditions that persist need to be treated by a physician.

Vitamins

Personally, I do not take vitamins or dietary supplements of any kind. When you are allowing your body to call for exactly what it needs, then it does not need to be fed artificial forms of those nutrients. Basically, there is no need to worry if you are getting vitamins. They are found everywhere—scattered all through foods. Many people eat cereal, toast, and orange juice for breakfast, and for a little insurance, they take a multipurpose vitamin pill. Let us take a look at this breakfast.

A typical cereal nowadays meets the U.S. RDA for vitamins and minerals. The U.S. RDA is a generous estimate of the protein, carbohydrate, fat, and minerals needs of a large, growing, teenage boy, who could possibly need 3,000–4,000 calories per day. In other words, these estimated needs would be way over what a grown five-foot, two-inch woman needs. So to even meet 100 percent of the U.S. RDA is overkill for most of our population.

God made cows' milk rich with nutrients. In addition, the government requires that we fortify milk with vitamins A and D, and perhaps some extra calcium, although milk happens to be *rich* in nutrients to start with. The piece of toast is enriched with niacin, thiamin, riboflavin, and iron. (Bread has been enriched this way since the 1930s.) These nutrients are also in the cereal and milk. The orange juice is high in vitamin C, as is the cereal, and nowadays it

might have extra calcium added to it. We now swallow a v
that meets the U.S. RDA (again, the needs of a growing teenage
and that is *breakfast!* If we are a five-foot, two-inch female, we mig
have met our personal nutrient needs by 500 percent or more for
some nutrients by 8 A.M.

Some people argue that vitamins (natural or synthetic) or herbs
are necessary for good health because the soil is depleted. This is
not true. When soil is depleted, it makes a smaller carrot than it would
if it were fertile. If you have two carrots—one from depleted soil
and one from fertile soil—the two carrots are the same chemically,
and thus have the same nutrients. Fertile soil would produce larger
and more carrots. If the soil were totally depleted, a carrot could not
be made. A cow grazing in a less fertile field will make less milk. But
milk is milk all across the country. Primarily, fertilizing increases
volume.

Some individuals have prescriptions for vitamins because they
have special conditions—usually malabsorption syndromes. Please
check with your physician. There is a need, however, to watch out
for overdosing on vitamins. Taking frequent, large doses of vitamins
is *not* natural, and since we are the first generation to do this, all of
the bad side effects are not yet known. I have had people that I counseled who had peripheral numbness (of their hands and feet). The
physicians diagnosed it as ten times the normal amount of vitamin
B_{12} in the bloodstream from taking prenatal vitamins for years. "If a
little is good—a lot is better." Wrong! Overdosing in small amounts
over time could be *very* bad for you.

Others have brought me sacks of vitamin pills that overlapped;
for example, vitamins C and E, multipurpose vitamins (more C and
E), and vitamin E. My suggestion is to slowly come back down off
this overdosing under a physician's monitoring. You will feel *so* much
better and have more money in your pocketbook.

Artificial sweeteners

As you have noticed, we suggest diet sodas and artificially sweetened tea. These noncaloric drinks may be used in place of sugared
beverages to help your blood sugar levels drop normally so that

WEIGH DOWN†

89

ct hunger. The artificial sweetener called as-
r fire in past years for allegedly causing side

the most thoroughly tested and screened
ket today. The Federal Food and Drug Ad-
﹍ ﹍ssued approval for aspartame twenty-six times.
﹍﹍﹍ American Council on Science and Health unequivocally en-
dorses its safety.

Aspartame is made up of two amino acids. An amino acid is just
one of the smallest units of a protein molecule. Many different amino
acids in different combinations make up the proteins you eat. The
amino acids in aspartame—phenylalanine and aspartic acid—are
found naturally in many foods. For example, if you eat a hamburger
patty, you will ingest much more aspartame than you would drink
from a two-liter bottle of diet soda. If you believe you get headaches
from diet sodas, and if the aspartame/headache theory is correct,
then you should get a migraine from one hamburger patty! However, research has shown no such adverse effects, even after repeated
double-blind, placebo-controlled clinical trials. One test done at Duke
University on people who claimed they experienced aspartame-in-
duced headaches showed the group who took aspartame actually
had *fewer* headaches than the control group who took placebos.

Headaches can be caused by many things, including stress and
sinus infections. (Even if you do not feel stuffy in your nose, the
sinus cavities could have a small infection that causes headaches.) It
could be that you are hungry. A diet drink should not give you a
headache because of a common protein molecule it contains. However, if you guzzle a cold drink too fast, then you might get a headache. Research currently being conducted is checking out other possible causes of these claims.

Saccharin, on the other hand, is different because it is a man-made
substitute. It is not found naturally in any foods and has caused
cancer in laboratory animals when given in very large doses. This
five-carbon unit is chemically similar to table sugar, but the tongue
and brain are not as easily fooled by this man-made sugar substitute. That is why it leaves a stronger aftertaste in your mouth. Saccharin has been banned in Europe for years. It has had the U.S. Sur-

geon General's warning on it since the 1970s: "Use of this product may be hazardous to your health. This product contains saccharin, which has been determined to cause cancer in laboratory animals."

Be slow to put your hope in food claims—that they cure you or harm you. There is so much conflicting evidence.

Placebo effects are powerful. A person who believes a pill will make him stronger or more healthy—or, vice versa, that a substance will harm him—will be affected by that belief.

One example I remember from years ago was where a very large study was done on the claim that vitamin C cured the common cold. A thousand people were put on vitamin C and another thousand were put on an orange powdered pill (a placebo). Not even the person or the interviewer knew who was on what so that they could not bias the report. The people with the lowest number of colds were on the placebo!

It is good to be wise regarding wellness claims made about specific foods these days. For example, government researchers might be a great resource for objective information about foods, whereas a food manufacturer might exaggerate its product's benefits for certain diseases or good health. A doctor selling pills or honey at his front counter might tend to exaggerate their medicinal benefits. Claims that certain food concoctions can cure cancer, arthritis, or headaches should be closely scrutinized. Just as you cannot swallow gelatin tablets (powder made from horses' hooves) and make this very incomplete protein go to your fingernails to strengthen them, you cannot make certain foods you eat directly affect some isolated cancer cells. Put your hope in God—not food concoctions. Believe me, if there were some foods that *cured* some disease, we would know about it. You could not stop that kind of news.

The point is to be slow to jump on the bandwagon. One month we hear that oatmeal is beneficial in lowering cholesterol, and the next month we find out that long-term research contradicts the short-term findings. Researchers may have stock in food industries, and pharmaceuticals all have vested financial interests in claiming certain findings, so be accurate with your volume of food and do not be overly optimistic with a food claim.

In conclusion, your body was made with great wisdom. You

mainly need to know *how much* food you need. That is the main sensitivity to good health. What you need is so overlapped in each food group that what you eat is not complicated or something to *worry* about. It is universally accepted to have breakfast foods that differ from lunch and supper foods in the course of one day. This familiar acceptance of variety lets you know that God has programmed our systems to have biological feedback that cues us to a variety, even within a twenty-four–hour period.

There are no "trigger foods" or foods that are capable of controlling you. You are free now to eat regular food the rest of your life. You will be in control and you will eat a variety. If you are not convinced, do this little experiment:

Try eating chocolate for breakfast, lunch and supper for several days in a row. Eat chocolate for breakfast while everyone else is eating buttered biscuits with eggs and bacon. Now, the next time you are hungry, you can eat chocolate while everyone else at the table is eating hamburgers and salty French fries. For supper, you eat chocolate again while everyone is eating salad with blue cheese dressing and grilled salmon. In my years of counselling, I have never known anyone who could desire only chocolate for three days in a row. On that routine, even the thought of chocolate will make you nauseated (biological feedback), you will have diarrhea (the body's way to try to protect you), and you may not desire chocolate again for weeks (biological feedback to protect you). *Wake up* and use your new internal control. You can do it!

To give you a better idea of the variety of food we are free to enjoy, I have included a typical three days' menu of my own on the facing page.

Remember, you are free from man-made rules. So you do not have to follow this menu; it is just an example. God may have created you to desire something totally different. Think about it: if He made us all have the same tastes in food, our favorite food would soon run out. Is He not a genius?

God intended for us to enjoy all foods. I love both broccoli and Häagen-Dazs ice cream, and I feel no guilt for whatever my body desires. I have been eating this way since 1978 and I am still in great health, with hard nails and healthy hair—all by following the inge-

Day one

Breakfast. . . . . Biscuit with butter and jelly, 1-3 slices of bacon, coffee with cream (depending on hunger level, some may be left over)

Lunch. . . . . Sandwich (white bread, ham, mayonnaise, lettuce), a few plain potato chips, small Snickers bar, diet soda (left some)

Afternoon. . . . . Diet soda

Supper. . . . . Lasagna, salad with blue cheese dressing, roll, lemon pie, unsweetened tea (left behind some of everything)

Nighttime snack. . . . Leftover slice of lemon pie, decaf coffee

Day two

Breakfast . . . . Cinnamon roll, coffee with cream

Lunch . . . . Sandwich (hoagie bun, roast beef, lettuce, tomato, mayonnaise), bag of barbecue potato chips, Danish wedding cookies (five in all, each one broken into smaller units and savored), diet soda (As usual, food remaining on the plate looked as if it had been dissected!)

Supper . . . . Chicken broccoli casserole, squash, roll, a few bites of pecan pie, unsweetened tea (picked over and the best eaten)

Nighttime snack. . . . Small bowl of cereal or fruit-flavored beverage

Day three

Breakfast , ... Cereal with milk, coffee with cream

Lunch . . . . Hamburger with all the fixings, a few french fries with ketchup, brownie, diet soda

Supper. . . . . Steak, most delectable portion of a baked potato with butter and sour cream, salad with blue cheese dressing, roll, pecan pie, milk (2 percent)

Nighttime snack. . . . not hungry—didn't think about food

Figure 8-4: Gwen's sample three days' menu. Her amounts vary according to her hunger. Don't use this as a guide for your own eating. The thousands of people in Weigh Down[†] have all eaten something different and have lost weight. Use your own hunger and preference to select your amounts and menus.

nious plan of God.

There is much confusion in regard to what gives you optimum health and longevity. Not many people can argue the fact that the single most related factor to longevity is thinness and, vice versa, the single most related factor to early death or accelerated aging is overeating. Medicine has advanced in many areas of treatment of certain diseases and yet has remained flat in others. Caution should be used in new and unfounded claims of food and its relation to cures of diseases. One thing is for sure—going to God is always good.

It is interesting to note that when people came to be healed from certain diseases in the Old and New Testaments, there was never a common denominator of what was done (dipping seven times in the Jordan River, a paste of spit and mud put on the eyes, touching the hem of Jesus' garment, etc.), but the common denominator was that they all went to the Father. We need to do the same.

How to Stop
When You Are Full

To start with, what in the world is the definition of *full?* I used to know no end to fullness. It seemed as if I could eat all day and not get full. I know that slightly full meant that I had to take off my belt, moderately full meant that I had to take off all my clothes and put on my robe, and painfully full meant that the only position I could get in was horizontal. Those are the full sensations, right? Well, not anymore. Full is a very polite feeling. In fact, when you are approaching fullness and you can still bend over and reach down and pick up your napkin off the floor without losing all your food, then you can be sure that you are not over full! It is also a good sign that you can leave your clothes on—especially your belt! If you think that you are having trouble with going beyond the polite full feeling, then maybe a few tips will help you.

The best advice is to *slow down* your eating until your heart's desire has changed so that it is repulsive and too painful to eat beyond full. The habit of eating fast developed as you became more magnetized to the refrigerator. It does not take food lovers long to learn that the faster they eat, the more food they can get down before it is too painful. This is a choice. Keep in mind, if you are having difficulty with stopping, perhaps it is because you have spent years obeying the food. Now is the time to reverse that behavior and take control over the food.

To help learn how to slow down, let us first look at *why* we should slow down. It seems that many of us have used poor role models for how we are to eat. The average meal is consumed inside three minutes. Let us just follow food through the digestive tract and see what happens when we eat very quickly.

Here are the major stops food takes on the way into the bloodstream. First, the food goes down your esophagus. As you swallow, two sets of muscles will push the food downward (peristalsis). This

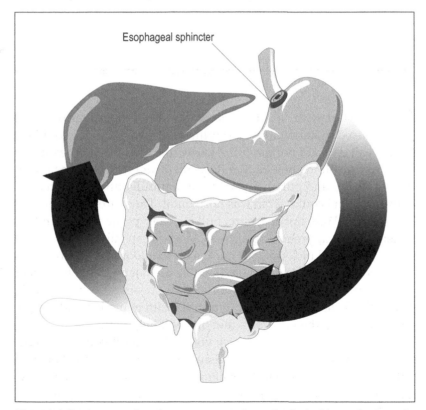

Figure 9-1: It takes approximately ten to twenty minutes for the food ingested to enter the bloodstream in the form of glucose and "turn off" the hunger feeling.

looks similar to the waves you see when a snake eats. At the base of the esophagus and stomach are sphincters. A sphincter is a circular ring of muscles that can close tightly. The esophageal sphincter regulates the passage of food through the upper digestive tract.

If you eat too fast, then you could possibly eat beyond fullness because your food has not had sufficient time to be digested and sent into the bloodstream. So—slow it down. Savor your food bite by bite.

Another problem you might encounter occurs when you eat only solid foods at the mealtime and then drink liquids afterwards. Keep in mind that your food must be diluted with water before your stomach can digest it. The more solids you eat, the more water the stomach needs. This fluid can come from the bloodstream or your thirst mechanism may cause you to drink more fluids.

The bottom line is that you need to drink or sip between bites. This really helps keep you from getting too full. You need to know that fatty foods will float to the top of the stomach, and their presence will slow down digestion. It takes approximately twenty minutes for the brain to detect the replenished blood sugar—but a skilled thin eater will notice a full stomach pouch and a decreased sensitivity to the flavor of the food.

When you develop your skills for recognizing the full feeling and stopping when you are full, you will be able to eat faster if you want to. You will learn to recognize when you are approaching full—even if you eat fast. Our goal is not to slow you down in eating—our goal is to help you to not stuff yourself. Once you lose the greed for food, we do not care how you eat. That is between you and your *mother!*

What happens when you frequently stuff the stomach? You get indigestion or heartburn or the acid refluxes into the esophagus. As we have said before, under normal conditions, food remains in the stomach until the acidity reaches a pH of 1.5. This is very acidic—much like battery acid. Then it will start to empty. The food will be allowed out of the stomach and into the small intestine. When you overload the stomach by eating too fast, your body is unable to manufacture enough neutralizing base to offset the extra acid the stomach produces to digest the extra food. That is why overeaters frequently get ulcers in the duodenum and heartburn in the esophagus. Acidic food literally refluxes out of both ends of the stomach, causing pain. Most people who faithfully start the Weigh Down Workshop† never have any more pain associated with eating!

Next the small, broken-down particles move through vessels to the liver. The liver is a chemical factory that is capable of turning what you eat into the substances your body needs. If you happen to swallow a trace amount of a chemical that the body does not like, such as a pesticide, then the liver traps it and breaks it down, preventing it from entering your normal bloodstream or damaging your liver. But the usable food particles are passed on by your liver to the heart, where they will be pumped all over the body.

Once the food particles enter the regular bloodstream, your feeling is one of fullness and satisfaction. Your stomach may feel full five minutes after a quick meal, but that truly satisfied feeling, which comes from nutrients hitting the normal bloodstream, may take another ten minutes.

Children digest food much faster than adults and feel like playing right after a meal. That is OK. Let them. However, when adults eat too much, they feel lethargic. Blood and water rush to the stomach to digest the huge amount of food. This leaves less blood for the brain and other parts of the body. It takes a lot of energy to digest huge meals, especially after overindulgence, since the food has to be converted to fats and shipped to the hips.

> Do not join those who drink too much wine
>   or gorge themselves on meat,
> for drunkards and gluttons become poor,
>   and drowsiness clothes them in rags. (Proverbs 23:20,21)

If you will eat smaller amounts, you will not have this problem. You will have less heartburn, fewer ulcers, and more energy.

Increased physiological hunger due to hormonal changes

Unfortunately, the increased hunger associated with a woman's monthly menstrual cycle has been greatly exaggerated to the point that it is just an invitation to gluttony for some. Yes, the body becomes slightly hungrier as it prepares itself to handle conception. However, what most do not realize is that once the body does not conceive and menses begins, a woman's hunger will drop back in proportion to the increased hunger beforehand. This decreasing hunger is the thing that no one seems to want to pick up on! Emotions are slightly more sensitive at some stages of the monthly cycle, but women should not run to food. We can have no more invitations to emotional eating.

Tips for slowing down

1. Pray for God to help you slow down and watch what happens. It will amaze you!
2. Try stopping in the middle of your meal for one to two minutes. Give the food time to hit the bloodstream and really satisfy your hunger.
3. Try drinking two or three ounces of orange juice or sweet beverage before you start. If you feel ravenous and too hungry, you may be afraid that you will never stop! By drinking a couple of ounces of juice before eating, you will quickly bring the blood sugar up enough to give you a calming effect that will allow you to approach the food with more control. This has helped some people.
4. Try looking up from the food. Enjoy the company. Have you ever been at a dinner where all you saw was the top of people's heads as they had their faces buried in their plates? It shows a lot of love and affection for that plate of food. Divorce yourself from that food! Sit up, talk to the people you are with, carry on some polite dinner conversation, and ask the kids how their day was at school. That is the very essence of the family dinner, to have the opportunity to spend time together interacting.
5. Try using a fork. Americans rarely use eating utensils these days. Look at a typical day in this country. You get up and have your cup of orange juice and a biscuit. Midmorning, you have coffee. At lunch, you have a sandwich and some chips. In the afternoon, you have an apple. At supper, you have pizza. Did you notice you did not use a single fork all day? Try using utensils again, even on something that you traditionally eat

with your hands. Cut up the pizza. It is a lot neater, and you will be able to make the bites smaller. That will slow you down.

6. Try sipping between bites. This will give you time between each bite and keep you from packing the next bite in on top of the one you have not finished savoring.

7. Try taking smaller bites. This will slow you down, and the pie will not be gone in four bites. Again, as we mentioned before with the forks, it will allow you to savor the food longer. One of the easiest ways to take smaller bites is to break up the food. For example, you can break chips or cookies into smaller bites rather than popping a whole one in your mouth. Try cutting up sandwiches and pizza.

8. Get the food out of your sight when you even suspect you are comfortably full. Cover up the plate with your napkin, push the plate an arm's length away, or better yet, leave the table and go into another room and pray for God to remove the desire to eat another bite. Give Him a few minutes, and He will answer the prayer. Sometimes He will answer before you finish your prayer. He is able to rescue you.

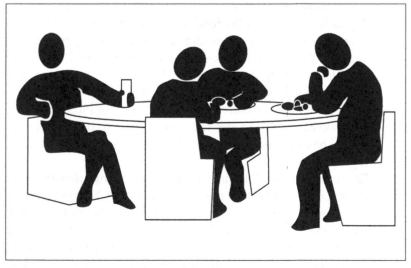

Figure 9-2: Try to raise your head out of the plate and look around and talk to people. Show less affection for the food. It's not your love anymore.

Slowing down could help your awareness of your stomach's getting full. The food entering the bloodstream will signal the hypothalamus to turn off hunger signals. Salivation decreases, as does stomach acid production, the sense of smell, and taste bud acuity.

Proverbs 27:7 says, "He who is full loathes honey, but to the hungry even what is bitter tastes sweet." It reflects the law of diminishing returns. When you are very hungry, God makes the tongue delight in the taste of the food. As you approach the point that the body is getting enough food (full), God makes your taste buds lose interest in the taste of the food, even sweet foods! The purpose is to help turn off the eating behavior. If you keep practicing, you will get better at knowing the difference between too full and comfortably full.

In the event that you are still fighting the battle of "But my mouth still wants some more," you should try to be creative. For example, you are eating lunch—say a submarine sandwich on a hoagie bun with sesame seeds on top. You feel the sensation that you are no longer hungry, but you would kind of like to keep going. Start dissecting the sandwich. Pull out small pinches of the meat you like the best, or the cheese you like the best, or the tasty pepper or olive. Slowly savor each small pinch, sipping between bites and even having a small sesame seed or two in between. You will still be with the company, but you will not really be consuming much food. Also, you still are getting little tastes until your "blood sugar full" signal clearly tells you that you have had enough. Then it will be easy for you to throw away the rest or save it for the next meal.

If you are having dessert, do the same thing. Just barely skim the edge of the lemon meringue pie onto your fork and savor the smallest amount. Nibble on the edges of your favorite cookie. Let paper-thin slices of chocolate melt in your mouth.

If you are eating out, you can always ask the server to bring a carryout container at the beginning of the meal. When your meal arrives, you can immediately put half of it in the container. This way you are putting the temptation out of your sight.

Let me give you another approach. You are at home and having family dinner. You are halfway through your serving of casserole when that feeling hits you that you are no longer hungry. Sometimes it will occur to you when you have only a bite or two left. Do not pop those last couple of bites into your mouth. Try this instead. Get up and walk away from the table for a few minutes. See if anyone else wants something to drink. This break buys you some time for your "blood sugar full" to register clearly so that you can come back to the table in a few minutes and feel the full feeling of nutrients in the bloodstream. It will now be easier to give those leftovers to the dog.

By the way, God made dogs to love humans' leftovers, perhaps so that we would not have so much garbage. I have the healthiest animals from this money-saving tip. The dogs and cats love it. If your dog is food-focused, just give it affection instead of food every time it wants more food than is needed, and the dog will lose interest in the food—the same principle as for people, and it works better than diet dog food!

How to stop bingeing or purging

First of all, understand that you do not have a disease and that you are not physiologically addicted to specific foods you binge on. For example, some diet counselors would have you believe that eating a simple carbohydrate will trigger an uncontrollable binge. That is not true.

There are addictions, however. It has been assumed all these years that addictions to tobacco, alcohol, drugs, or caffeine are *only* physiological and psychological. It is a fact that alcoholics will sometimes experience delirium tremens when deprived of alcohol. But reconsider for one moment. The body compensates the best it can to accommodate carbon monoxide, or extra food, or anything else that is harmful. But the body welcomes the reversal of harmful habits. In other words, your lungs do not want more smoke. Your thighs do not want more fat. The liver does not want more alcohol.

We propose, rather, the majority of the addiction is a heart, or spiritual, addiction. Withdrawals are, equally, the product of the feeling of the separation of your heart from loving the substance. It is analogous to trying to take a fifteen-month-old out of the arms of its mother. Your dependent spirit is addicted to the love of the sub-

stance, and letting go of food or tobacco will really be hard and emotionally difficult unless you simultaneously replace that dependence
with clinging onto God. People who have been addicted to drugs
for 30 years have had the experience of finding God and the accom-
panying ability to stop using the drugs. In the case of food, we believe that it is only a spiritual addiction. Years of dieting breeds the
"starve-binge-purge" cycle.

You want to lose weight. You start a diet, starving yourself of both
calories and the foods you like. When you reach the point that you
cannot take it anymore, you throw in the towel and binge. You feel
guilty for the binge, so you purge to correct the binge.

The purge is an attempt on your part to eliminate from your system the calories that you took in from the binge or food that you
have been led to believe is "bad for you" or "too high in fat." Purging takes many forms. Some examples are vomiting (bulimia), fluid
pills (diuretics), laxatives, or exercise. Do you not see that all of these
actions are the results of your trying to fix everything? Your path is
destructive, and with every step you take, you are forced to try to
undo what you just did. And what you just did was supposed to
have been the solution. Every step made it worse!

So what *is* the root of the problem? It is what your heart is depending on! Bingeing is not a separate phenomenon. If certain foods
seem to trigger the invitation to binge, again it is not a physiological
addiction, but rather, a spiritual dependency on these foods for comfort and love. It is not an addiction to sugar or fat. And purging is
not some disease or obsession. It is all a consequence of your lust for
food. From that perspective, here is the cycle:

You have a passion for food rather than God. That passion for
food leads to overeating. Overeating leads to overweight. Overweight leads to dieting. Dieting does not address your misplaced
passion, and deprivation while on this diet explodes in a binge. The
ensuing guilt can take you in two directions:

1. You can repent (turn back to God), ask for His help, and sim-
    ply wait until your body empties again. You may feel too full,
    and it may take a while before you feel hunger again, but do
    not worry—you will be fine. You must practice being depen-
    dent on God. If you call out to God, He can give you the peace

you need and the control feeling you are looking for—with no
guilt. In other words, God can make you feel better than purging.
2. Or you can bypass God, try by your own power to correct the
mess you have made, and take the purging route. This second
option is obviously never-ending because it does not address
or uproot the lust for food.

The way to end the entire cycle is to transfer your passion for food
to passion for God. What the diet industry has done in this country
has resulted in years and years of deprivation from man-made rules.
The deprivation that I am referring to is of two basic forms. It is
either a caloric deprivation (for example, counting calories every
day) or food category deprivation (for example, no sugars or fats).
Caloric deprivation causes you to starve off the fat until you just
cannot take it anymore. You then eat everything in sight. Americans
have been known to consume thousands of calories in binges.

The second area of deprivation that we can address is caused by
the prolonged abstinence from certain food groups. Typically, the
average weight-reduction diet eliminates sweets and fats, and some
eliminate all sugars, flour, and so on. This constant refusal to give
the body a nutrient it is calling for will ultimately result in a binge.
The secret rendezvous at the candy store or bakery, with destruction of the wrappers so no evidence will be found, ends with the
ensuing guilty feeling of having cheated and deceived; but the rules
you break are man's, not God's. So the resulting guilt is false guilt.

You punish yourself with a good long fast—that is, more deprivation—to get the extra calories out of your system. After years of
purging, some people seem to automatically throw up after a meal.
This is reverse peristalsis. Just don't worry about it—your body is
confused now, but it will settle back down to normal forward-mov-
ing peristalsis.

Some of you have spent years in therapy trying to combat the
false guilt and to treat your obsessive behavior. Obsessive behavior
includes excessive exercise, starvation diets, or consumption of laxatives. Please relax—God can help you through this.

Bulimia, or purging, is what I call a second-generation disorder.
You saw your mother or father overeat and then try to solve their

problem with a diet sheet. They only got bigger, so you (the next generation) got smart (?) and said, "Diets are not really working, so I will throw it up (purge) or take a laxative."

Let me tell you right now that you can be set free from all of that behavior. Let us not band-aid the symptom, though; let us go straight to the root. The Weigh Down Workshop[†] approach to eating is absolutely the answer to it all. Both generations chose not to eat less food. Here is the way to break the cycle:

1. Stop dieting and starving or purging to fix the binge or any overeating. Replace it with hunger and fullness living. The result will be no deprivation as you wake up today and know that as soon as you get hungry, you will be able to eat.

2. Replace the intensive desire to eat with an intensive desire for God, and the bingeing will end. As a result, the bulimia will subside.

Now that a solution is given—hunger and fullness—purging is no longer necessary, and purging episodes will subside.

So you can see the binge is not caused by an "addiction" to sugar or chocolate. We are emphatically telling you that you can eat whatever your body is calling for and that you do not have to make the food righteous ever again. Do not be afraid of the fats and sugars. You are not addicted to them; you just want them excessively because you have not been allowed to have them for so long.

It is like Eve in the Garden; those foods are forbidden fruit, and as soon as they are put into that category, then they will be exactly what you want the most. By reintroducing yourself to these foods, you will not only learn to eat them with control, but also many of these so-called "forbidden fruits" will lose their appeal after a while.

A certain sense of peace comes with knowing that whenever you get hungry, you may have that food. Again, as we have stated before, your body has incredible biological feedback for variety. Once you have had enough of that one food, you will not want it again for a while.

Don't be afraid, however, if that "while" seems to take longer than you thought it should. You may have literally years of deprivation to erase. Soon you will begin to sense that your body is calling for many other foods, and you can begin to freely eat more of a variety.

Tips for your heart

This chapter is a tough chapter because it is a telling chapter. Some of these tips may or may not help you. You may want to ask God to give you some tips that will help you personally. However, if your heart does not want to stop when you are full and it wants to eat everything on the plate and it would really like what is left over on the children's plates, then stopping tips are not what you need right now. You need a few heart tips.

Why in the world would we ever want more than we need? Why would we ever try to override our body's controls on the amount of food we eat? I think it is a pretty easy answer. We feel that we need to take care of ourselves because no one else in this world will care about us. We eat as if there is no tomorrow, thinking we had better "get while the getting is good." Perhaps we are not so sure that we believe there is a God, especially a caring Father/Creator. We do not know God's personality well enough to know that He likes burrito supremes with extra sour cream. He wants us to taste and enjoy all kinds of foods, especially desserts, all of our lives. However, He wants to be the provider or the one to indulge us. And yet, we indulge ourselves so much that we do not even give God a chance. He would like us to wait for hunger so He can delight us with the new Mexican restaurant for supper—but He cannot, because we carved ourselves out a pan of brownies and bowed down to it earlier in the afternoon. We decided on our indulgence, cooked it, and ate it. God gets squeezed out of our lives as we refuse to wait on Him or look to Him.

This attitude is not new; the Israelites did the same thing when they grew impatient for Moses to bring God's laws to them.

> When the people saw that Moses was so long in coming down from the mountain, they gathered around Aaron and said, "Come, make us gods who will go before us. As for this fellow Moses who brought us up out of Egypt, we don't know what has happened to him."
>
> Aaron answered them, "Take off the gold earrings that your wives, your sons and your daughters are wearing, and bring them to me." So all the people took off their earrings and brought

them to Aaron. He took what they handed him and made it into
an idol cast in the shape of a calf, fashioning it with a tool. Then
they said, "These are your gods, O Israel, who brought you up
out of Egypt." (Exodus 32:1–4)
The Israelites, despite seeing all the ways God had provided for them,
created a false god to which they turned for comfort—to their ultimate sorrow.

What is more, we never get to thank Him because "We took care
of everything!" It is as if we are saying that we do not need God. I
would die right now if my children told me that they did not need
me anymore. I love to be needed and God loves it, too. The irony is
that we are desperate for Him and His loving, giving, and guiding
hand, and we hardly even know it!

If your heart only knew that God is going to let you get hungry
again and that He is going to feed you again! He is a great shepherd
who loves to feed His sheep physically and spiritually. In fact, the
picture of a shepherd is one who spends all day looking for a great
place for the sheep to feed. Look to Him for guidance about when to
start eating and when to stop. Believe Him when He says, "And
without faith it is impossible to please God, because anyone who
comes to him must believe that he exists and that he *rewards* those
who earnestly seek him" (Hebrews 11:6). You have got to come to
know how good He will be to you if you seek Him. If you will obey
God and not overindulge, there will be some reward for you. We
call these little rewards or happies from God *jewels*. So heart, cheer
up! A jewel will always be waiting for you if you stop when you are
full! One of the most important assignments in Weigh Down[†] is to
look for and find the jewels that God has given you.

We would like to stress the importance of stopping at the earliest
signals of being physiologically full. But if your longing heart is still
yearning, food will not satisfy it. It would be great to finish each
evening meal by taking a walk around the block—just you and the
Lord. Give Him your broken heart and problems. He will fix those.
Just obey Him with your food.

Pray that your *desire* to eat slows down. It is all a matter of your
heart. If your heart loses its desire for food, eating slowly is a breeze,
and going beyond full is out of the question.

HOW TO EAT POTATO CHIPS
AND CHOCOLATE

We are the salt of the earth, according to Matthew 5:13. This used to be a compliment to people. It meant that they added flavor and enhanced the world around them. Now that salt has been on the hit list for the last two decades, that scripture has lost its meaning. Well, you probably know how I feel about salt by now. I thank our good Lord above for the spectacular creation of sodium chloride—table salt. I love salt. Cows go up to salt licks, and animals will use the natural salt licks in the wild all summer long.

I get in the mood for a salt lick every once in a while. What I do is get a bowl of Mexican chips with a tomato-based salsa. I will hold every chip up to the light to see if it sparkles. If it sparkles, that chip has a lot of salt on it. I used to try to do this at the restaurant when no one was looking—now I do not care! After examining several chips, I usually find one. Great! Now I will dip it into the salsa, and sometimes I have been known to add even more salt to the top of that. Oh, how fun that is with a diet soda going down between the bites! I am a double-dipper. I have to have my own salsa bowl because I never cram down one whole chip. I just eat small but perfect bites. Sometimes I am so full from the appetizer that I can only eat a few bites of my chicken quesadilla entrée with sour cream and guacamole on each bite.

You have to know what you are craving. If you are craving some salt, please do not go through stacks of unsalted chips or piles of slightly salted chips to find your salt. Purchase the saltiest of chips. I feel sorry for the food manufacturers. Just about the time they have changed the production lines to lower the salt and lower the fat content, people like us put salt and fat back in vogue—and the consumer demands that the manufacturer change the food again!

As long as you are eating when you are hungry and stopping when you are full and you have healthy kidneys (their job is to eliminate extra salt in the body), your blood pressure will normally not be affected by table salt (NaCl). The reason health professionals had to pull out the sugar, salt, and fat from the typical American diet was because of the ever-increasing volumes of food we were eating. To satisfy Americans' desire to swallow more food without increasing their calories, the food manufacturers had to pull out almost everything from the food but fiber and air. When you are overweight, it is harder for your kidneys to work properly and for the blood to circulate due to pressure from the surrounding layers of fat. This is especially true when the overweight person sits a lot. The sitting position inhibits blood flow for the overweight person. Salt may accumulate in blood and move out of the vessels between the cells. Fluid retention that causes edema or swelling follows. Now that we are being reasonable in the volume we are swallowing, the content selection can be rich and delectable!

What about sweets? Make sure you go back and really rate the sweets you are eating. Get only the best. To help you learn to eat sweets again, we are going to start you with chocolates in small units. A good example of chocolate already in small units is M&Ms. Now, instead of ripping off the top of the package and then throwing your head back and dumping the M&Ms down the hatch,

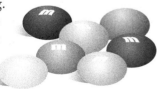

Figure 10-1: Let M&Ms melt in your mouth and not in your tummy. Your stomach cannot taste anything!

tear off the top of the package, stick your finger down in the package, and wiggle up one at a time. Of course, you may lose your grip and have to start over. You may get your least-favorite color and have to throw it back into the pile and start again. (You must rate your foods, you know.) But I feel certain you will eventually manage to get an M&M into your hand.

Now you need to put just one M&M into your mouth and let it melt in your mouth and not in your tummy. Your stomach cannot taste. I have a real ritual with M&Ms. I will let the M&M sit on my tongue until the candy coating is off. Then when I feel it is really thin, I crush the shell with the top of my mouth and all the melted milk chocolate comes out. Of course, I sip something hot between the bites of almost all sweets I eat. My coffee with real half-and-half cream helps to wash off the overly sweet taste, and then I am ready for another M&M. You are not going to get a lot of M&Ms down that way! Sometimes five or six will satisfy. Keep practicing with small units at the end of the meal.

Most of the world—in fact, probably all of the world's populations—offers dessert at the end of the meal. God created man to like this or how would so many diverse populations do the same thing? I have noticed my own cravings as I get toward the end of a meal. This same feeling comes over me: *"I'm nearly finished, so give me my dessert or sweet."* Dessert just indicates the end of eating. It pacifies me and concludes the eating event. My servings are small and I take small bites, savoring every bite, and I drink between bites. Yum! But I quit when I am politely full.

If you are still having trouble with overwhelming magnetism for the salts and sweets, hang on. Phase II will help you turn that around. As you open up each page of Phase II, God will make you face some tough things about yourself. Do not fear, for you will find that it won't be with dread, but almost with anticipation as you progressively make this transfer from love of food to love of God!

PHASE II

I have indeed seen the oppression of my people in Egypt. I have heard their groaning and have come down to set them free.

—Acts 7:34

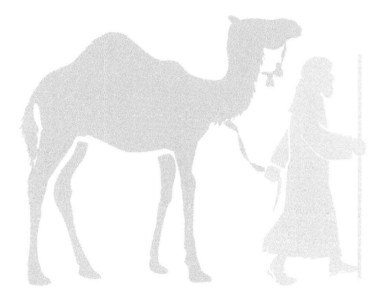

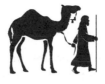

OUT OF EGYPT

*"Therefore I am now going to allure her; I will lead
her into the desert and speak tenderly to her."*
(God talking to the children of Israel, Hosea 2:14)

Y ou are entering Phase II of this journey. In this second phase
you will find yourself coming out of Egypt and entering
the Desert of Testing. I hope to give direction that will keep
you out of harm's way and away from desert storms and sand pits.

The concepts I lay before you are simple. They are so simple that
they will confound the intellectual elite. The intent of this book was
never to be a thorough scholarly explanation of Scripture to prove
points that have been debated by theologians for hundreds of years.
I would have to write volumes to build a logical basis of scriptural
references to prove something to debaters. That is not my intent.

This book is written for those who want to live out the truth. Those
of you who try to incorporate the truths set before you will find out
if they are genuine or not. This has always been the barometer in my
life: if a principle is from God, it will bear fruit. It will give you peace
that is virtually free of anger, and it will liberate you from compulsive behaviors. You will ultimately feel a deep, loving nature per-
meating your soul, in contrast to an unloving nature at the root and
base of your soul.

Look for the fruit

Some people enjoy scholarly debates and arguments. But the Bible states we should stay away from arguments and look for the fruits of the teaching. The blind receiving sight and the crippled receiving the ability to walk were evidences Jesus used to show that the Almighty God was behind what He was doing. Likewise, the fruit found in others' lives, which comes from adopting these fresh but timeless principles, is the only reference or recommendation we use in the Weigh Down Workshop*. "Watch out for false prophets. They come to you in sheep's clothing, but inwardly they are ferocious wolves. By their fruit you will recognize them. Do people pick grapes from thornbushes, or figs from thistles? Likewise every good tree bears good fruit, but a bad tree bears bad fruit" (Matthew 7:15–17).

If you choose to try what we are suggesting, you will know immediately if it is truth or not. On the other hand, there are those who do not want to find God. They will argue with the validity of the very obvious and extraordinary fruit of deliverance and change in the lives of people in the Weigh Down Workshop*. Stay focused on the results.

Jesus made the blind see, and Bible teachers of the day still argued that His message was not from God.

Jesus answered, "My teaching is not my own. It comes from him who sent me. If anyone chooses to do God's will, he will find out whether my teaching comes from God or whether I speak on my own." (John 7:16,17)

Most of us have lived long enough to know that if you have been delivered from compulsive behaviors and you now "get it" (you were blind, but now you see), and suddenly you read the Old and New Testaments with understanding, then God has to be involved. In other words, most people recognize that it has to be attributed to God's truths, for only God could have saved them from entrenched overeating, drug dependence, and depression. These are not small matters. We are talking about prisoners unchained and captives set free, broken hearts that no bypass operation could remedy, being restored. This is bigger than the Berlin Wall coming down. It will be very hard to keep this kind of rescue quiet across the world.

Yes, the rescue is from God, and the rescuer, Jesus, was foretold by Isaiah hundreds of years before Jesus walked on the earth.

The Spirit of the Sovereign LORD is on me, because the LORD has anointed me to preach good news to the poor. He has sent me to bind up the brokenhearted, to proclaim freedom for the captives and release from darkness for the prisoners, to proclaim the year of the LORD's favor and the day of vengeance of our God, to comfort all who mourn, and provide for those who grieve in Zion— to bestow on them a crown of beauty instead of ashes, the oil of gladness instead of mourning, and a garment of praise instead of a spirit of despair [depression]. They will be called oaks of righteousness, a planting of the LORD for the display of his splendor. (Isaiah 61:1–3)

What a beautiful picture of what is happening to you right now! Look at the fruit in your life from living these truths, or just look at where you once were and where you have come. You have just been delivered from the clutches of the mighty Pharaoh, and you have been led across the Red Sea by the hand of God. Many of you have tried everything to escape the prison of dieting and the pain of overweight and now are joining a great exodus of people finally turning to God for His mighty rescue.

Just as the Israelites were set free from Egypt, you have just been set free to love God instead of the refrigerator or pantry. You have just been set free from making bricks for Pharaoh (dieting, counting fat grams, have-to exercising, pills, liquid fasts, foods you do not want to eat, constant weighing, clothes that do not fit, and the scorn of men, _____ . . . you fill in the blanks). The exciting thing is that you have found yourself doing "self-controlled" things that you have never done before, such as leaving food on your plate, eating regular food, forgetting that it is lunchtime and, at the same time, finding yourself interested in learning more about God and communicating with Him. You surely have been rescued! But this is a journey. Just as Scripture says: "Therefore, my dear friends, as you have always obeyed—not only in my presence, but now much more in my absence—continue to work out your salvation with fear and trembling, for it is God who works in you to will and to act according to his good purpose" (Philippians 2:12,13).

We need to continue to work out this salvation, to put off the old way of living and to put on the new. To do this requires your heart. Eventually, there will be an end to major battles with food or whatever you are working on with the Father.

As we have just described, you have already felt a difference in that your heart is pulled less by the refrigerator. You feel that one day you can walk away from your old love, food, and into the arms of the Father. But you have some distance to go before you get to the point that your heart has no desire to turn to food for comfort or for delight. In other words, you have some distance to go before your heart has been thoroughly tested. My prayer for you is: "Godspeed through the Desert of Testing to the Promised Land."

I personally was not desert-ready; I was unprepared for sandstorms, desert vipers, and hot temperatures. I hope that the words on these pages and in the following chapters of Phase II will help to make your journey a little easier. The Israelites took forty years to get to the Promised Land!

According to the map, a trip by foot from Egypt to the Promised Land should take only one or two weeks. But God was going to have to teach the Israelites some very important lessons first. He used the hot desert to strip them down to nothing so they could see what was in their hearts. From Egypt, they were led to the Desert of Sinai, or what I refer to as

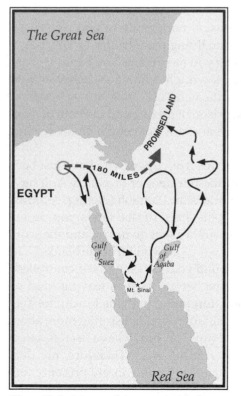

Figure 11-1: A two-week journey stretched over forty years while God taught Israel what He wanted them to know.

the *Desert of Testing*. The following chapters will help you along through the wilderness. Look at each of the following chapters like one desert oasis after another, a cool drink of water on your desert path.

God's passion for you

The first oasis we will bring you to is the subject of God's passion for you. This first bit of information is more like a bucket of water. It is foundational for making it through the Desert of Testing. Think of it as the water the camel stores to help him through the long dry spells in the desert. This first draw of water is the subject of God's love for you. We have talked continually of the need for you to love the Father, but does He really care about you? Yes, powerfully so! He does not allow your idols to save you, and He is waiting patiently to save you with His power when you finally call on Him. Next, He woos and courts you to be in His presence to be alone with Him in the desert. It is actually romantic.

Logically, it makes sense that He loves us. He has made us and loves us—just as we love our own cooking better than someone else's, or that the child "we made" is better than other children. In the same way, our maker is crazy about us. After all, He picked out everything: personality, hair color, handwriting style, eye color, birth date, environmental setting, and so on. He knows the food we like and has been trying to show us His love, and He has been patiently waiting for us to return it. We just need to open our eyes.

I could list a hundred scriptures that tell us that He loves us—but I know we want something we can feel and touch in order to know that He loves us. We want some concrete evidence.

The images that God uses to illustrate His emotion for us covers the spectrum. He uses father, mother, Jesus as our brother, and the Holy Spirit as a counselor. He talks about gathering us all in like a mother hen puts her wings around her little chicks. He is the very gentle, loving, patient Shepherd of the dependent sheep. He is the generous Father that gives the prodigal son all of his inheritance with no strings attached and waits longingly for him daily. He cares.

All of these are loving images. But the most moving is the passionate lover image of jealousy. Exodus 34:14 says, "Do not worship any other god, for the LORD, whose name is Jealous, is a jealous God."

So God is jealous for your attention and love. Did you know God loves you personally and individually and wants a covenant relationship with you? A covenant relationship is like a marriage. The word *covenant* means an arrangement made by one party that the other party could accept or reject but could not alter. He wants to marry you—or put another way, wants to marry your heart and soul. Jesus refers to the church as His bride. Take a look at an allegory in which Jerusalem (God's beloved) is represented first as a baby and then as a lover:

" 'On the day you were born your cord was not cut, nor were you washed with water to make you clean, nor were you rubbed with salt or wrapped in cloths. No one looked on you with pity or had compassion enough to do any of these things for you. Rather, you were thrown out into the open field, for on the day you were born you were despised.

" 'Then I passed by and saw you kicking about in your blood, and as you lay there in your blood I said to you, "Live!" I made you grow like a plant of the field. You grew up and developed and became the most beautiful of jewels. Your breasts were formed and your hair grew, you who were naked and bare.

" 'Later I passed by, and when I looked at you and saw that you were old enough for love, I spread the corner of my garment over you and covered your nakedness. I gave you my solemn oath and entered into a covenant with you, declares the Sovereign LORD, and you became mine.

" 'I bathed you with water and washed the blood from you and put ointments on you. I clothed you with an embroidered dress and put leather sandals on you. I dressed you in fine linen and covered you with costly garments. I adorned you with jewelry: I put bracelets on your arms and a necklace around your neck, and I put a ring on your nose, earrings on your ears and a beautiful crown on your head. So you were adorned with gold and silver; your clothes were of fine linen and costly fabric and embroidered cloth. Your food was fine flour, honey and olive oil. You became very beautiful and rose to be a queen. And your fame spread among the nations on account of your beauty, because the splendor I had given you made your beauty perfect, declares the Sovereign LORD.' " (Ezekiel 16:4–14)

This scripture leaves no doubt that God adores you and His church and wants an intimate relationship with you. It is like a husband and wife relationship. Christ is the bridegroom of the church, and He gave His own life for His bride.

There is more imagery. We have heard that God loved us so much that He gave His only Son to die on the cross. We have heard it so often that it conjures up very little emotion anymore. But if we have lost a child or know someone who has, or if we have personally experienced a kidnapping or watched our child in the emergency room or hospital bed, then it brings it home a little bit more. Losing a child is by far the most devastating of all crises—to lose one in whom you have invested your heart and soul and mind and strength. The idea of God sacrificing His own child for us to be able to have a love relationship with Him is just incredible!

Just as the parent loves the child more than the child loves the parent—God loves you more than you love Him. He loved first. Look at this passage from 1 John 4:7–10: "Dear friends, let us love one another, for love comes from God. Everyone who loves has been born of God and knows God. Whoever does not love does not know God, because God is love. This is how God showed his love among us: He sent His one and only Son into the world that we might live through him. This is love: not that we loved God, but that he loved us and sent his Son as an atoning sacrifice for our sins." We love ourselves—but we love our children even more. How many times have we sat by the bedside of our sick child and asked God to take out that sickness or infirmity and put it in our own body? We would rather die than see our child die. God could have shown His love by giving His own body—but a greater love is giving the life of His child to get to us. There is no greater way to symbolize how deeply He wants to draw us to Him.

Practical examples of God's attention and love

God does love us so much, and we are not alone. God is right there with us at all times. Even though you might think you are far apart, He is always in your heart. Recently, as I was driving to work, I worried that God was mad at me or that He was not "with me." So I pouted to Him and explained to Him that I had kept my end of the bargain and that I could feel the love I had for Him in my heart. It was a strong love. So I asked for something visible from this invisible God to show me that He was still there with me and loved me. I really could not come up with a creative sign for God, so I prayed that He would just send maybe a bird into view. Well, before the words got out of my mouth, I came upon a mail box that I had passed every day on my way to work. That day, the dove and the word "Faith" on the mail box jumped out at me.

God was telling me to have faith that He loves me. I started crying as I saw how kind He was to hear my prayers and answer them so quickly. All logical evidence shows that He is keeping His end of the "marriage" covenant relationship.

Physical reassurance builds our faith. I have never found God to get upset when we ask for evidence of His love; however, scriptures indicate that God does not like unbelievers to keep asking for signs to prove His existence (Matthew 16:1–4). How annoying that must be to God. We see the stars, His handiwork, His sunsets that have a different color scheme daily, and we witness the birth of new life. Yet some still demand a miraculous sign to prove the existence of God. Please! The writer of Romans put it this way: "The wrath of God is being revealed from heaven against all the godlessness and wickedness of men who suppress the truth by their wickedness, since what may be known about God is plain to them, because God has made it plain to them. For since the creation of the world God's invisible qualities —his eternal power and divine nature —have been clearly seen, being understood from what has been made, so that men are without excuse" (Romans 1:18–20).

God is tired of showing off in such fantastic ways and having people still demand a sign to prove His existence. But for the person pursuing a loving relationship with God, He provides whatever it takes to make His beloved secure in His presence. Asking for reassurance from God is not *testing* God—it is *seeking* God. That is His command for us.

Asking for reassurance from God is not testing God—it is seeking God. That is His command for us.

There are some who think, "Well, that is great for you. But God does not like 'lowlife' people like me." The Apostle Paul killed and imprisoned many people. But he turned to the Father, then turned out to be one of God's favorite people. The Samaritan woman at the well (John 4:4–28) had been married five times and was living with a sixth man; yet, Jesus showed compassion for her. Let me know if you have done worse than murdering a lot of people or are on your seventh marriage. You cannot mess up badly enough to stop the love God has for you.

In my seminars, I tell people who are feeling low or rejected or separated from the love of the Father to do just that. Ask for a sign of His personal love. Once again—try out these truths and see if what I am saying is from God! God will bring to your mind a fleece or sign to look for. One preacher wrote to me and said that he took me up on it. Take a look at what he found:

Dear Gwen,

As I drove to a friend's house for lunch today, I listened to your tape, "Beyond the Jordan." My family has been struggling for the last two years through some very dark and difficult times. Our faith has been greatly tested (and at times our marriage, too). At times my soul has felt barren and God's presence distant. We have wondered, "Will this ever pass?" Weigh Down has been an answer to prayer.

Today, while I was listening to a Weigh Down tape in the car,
you said, "Ask God for a sign of His presence." As I entered the
subdivision, a huge flock of blackbirds lifted off yet another blan-
ket of thick white snow. I thought to myself, "OK, Lord, we've
got plenty of blackbirds, hundreds of them; give me a cardinal . . . . No, make that a bluebird . . . . No, God, if You are truly
there, if You are still with me, give me both birds . . . *together.*"

After visiting awhile, my friend and I sat down for lunch. Right
in the middle of our meal I glanced out the window and almost
came unglued! I literally shouted, "Oh, my gosh!"

My friend said, "What, have you had a vision or something?"

Indeed, I had. For there, outside her window, seemingly having lunch together themselves, sat a cardinal and a bluebird on
the same bird feeder. It was not even thirty minutes after I had
asked God to give me a sign of His presence.

God is good . . . He is faithful . . . He is the jewel-giver. There *is*
hope.

Richard Ryan, Indiana

There is nothing more fun in life than looking for the attention and
personal love of the Father. He doesn't always use birds; He is waiting to "show off" His love and character to us in totally fresh and
unique ways. He is such a genius! It would bore Him to be anything
but incredible and mysterious in all of His ways. In Weigh Down[†],
we call the gifts and signs of His love *jewels,* and they are as numer-
ous as the sands on the seashore. We will report on jewels from God
in each of the following chapters. Start looking for your own.

When Satan comes in and tries to lie to you, telling you God is too
important and busy for the details of your life, just remember the
following story. One day I was outside sitting still. Some sparrows
lined up on a low roof edge. The first sparrow suddenly spread his
wings and flew down so fast, it looked like he "fell" to the ground.
The rest of the sparrows dropped to the ground one at a time in the
same fashion. I looked up to heaven and asked, "Oh Father, so that
is what you meant when Jesus said, 'Are not two sparrows sold for
a penny? Yet not one of them will *fall* to the ground apart from the
will of your Father' " (Matthew 10:29).

That day I felt I had more Scripture to back up what I already believed about the attentiveness of God. He knows not only when a sparrow falls down, gets hurt, or dies, but perhaps not one of the sparrows will "dive" to the ground without the Father's knowing about it! He knows when they are coming and going. How much more attentive He is to us, because we are His precious lambs. He loves us so much that He is just like parents who want to know where their teenagers are going and when they are coming home! God is even more interested than that! It is almost impossible for our hearts to comprehend this kind of attention. We are not used to it, but we need it.

"And even the very hairs of your head are all numbered. So don't be afraid; *you are worth more than many sparrows.*" (Matthew 10:30,31)

In other words, do not be afraid. He loves you and knows you so intimately that He has counted the hairs on your head. He has a digit assigned to each hair! He knows when one falls out! He knows you better than you know yourself!

. . . I pray that you, being rooted and established in love, may have power, together with all the saints, to grasp how wide and long and high and deep is the love of Christ, and to know this love that surpasses knowledge —that you may be filled to the measure of all the fullness of God. (Ephesians 3:17b–19)

I am absolutely delighting in exploring the boundaries of His love. I have not reached the edge of the width or the length, nor have I experienced the height or depth. Have faith and start looking for this love. If you have already found it, then there are still more surprises ahead for you. Just as love between a man and woman will result in the conception and birth of a life, this love of God to you will spring forth life in you.

So, God has called you. Now, follow Him into the desert.

"Therefore I am now going to allure her; I will lead her into the desert and speak tenderly to her. There I will give her back her vineyards, and will make the Valley of Trouble a door of hope. There she will sing as in the days of her youth, as in the day she came up out of Egypt." (Hosea 2:14,15)

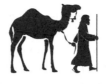

RISE ABOVE

Love the Lord with all of your mind . . .

Are you ready for another drink of cool water? In Phase I, you were presented with the picture of the *thin eater* or the person who feels no magnetic pull to food. We studied the externals—their behavior. But what in the world are they *thinking?* What is inside the brain of these rare creatures? Surely they have irregular brain waves; otherwise, how could they "waste" food? We have been told that we need to turn away from the refrigerator. But just exactly how are we supposed to accomplish this feat!? Why are others able to go through the buffet lines and remain in control while we feel like breaking the lines and eating everything in sight? Why do we feel out of control to the point that we avoid social events?

What is this compulsion called "desire eating?"

There is an explanation and a way out of compulsive and addictive behaviors. When Jesus said to love God with all of your heart, soul, mind, and strength and love your neighbor as yourself, that basically sums up all of Scripture. Do you realize how amazing that is? We can take thousands of words and phrases in the Old and New

Testament and sum them up in this passage in Mark that Jesus quoted from Deuteronomy:

> "The most important one," answered Jesus, "is this: 'Hear, O Israel, the Lord our God, the Lord is one. Love the Lord your God with all your heart and with all your soul and with all your mind and with all your strength.' " (Mark 12:29b,30)

We are going to take that scripture and break it down into its components. In this chapter we will start with the mind because it is one of the keys to rising above the magnetic pull of food.

Think about all the times over the years when an overwhelming urge came over you and you seemingly could not stop yourself from going to the refrigerator. Where in the world did that desire eating come from? And why does the *thin eater* not have it? What is the force or compulsion we were dealing with?

Most of the world does not give this question a whole lot of thought. The world has conveniently renamed this whole scene as simply an old habit. Is that not a nice, proper, non-convicting, sanitizing name for something that should really sound off an alarm bell in our hearts and in our heads?

This magnetic force toward food is a lot like the gravitational force that we have toward the earth. If you lose your footing, you will fall to the ground, right? That will never change. Gravity was a hard concept to learn; yet bumps, knocks, and bruises pounded the fact of gravity into your brain early in life. Now you understand that fact; you accept it and you work around it on a daily basis. You have long forgotten the pain of falling down the steps. Now, without having to think about it, you do what is necessary to avoid any problems with gravity. The force of gravity remains, but you have conquered it, so to speak.

The gravitational force toward the things of this world is also out there. It has been around for a long, long time. Whether you have paid any attention to it does not change the reality of its presence. You can call it a habit and ignore it if you want to. However, you must think this through to be able to rise above the force of any of the world's allures.

How to conquer eating compulsions

Some people do not know that God can help them conquer the pull of the pantry. In the past, many skeptics did not believe we could conquer gravitational forces, either. We enjoy modern airplanes today, thanks to the aviators who went against all earthly reason and suffered man's scorn for their early failures, but who finally achieved manned flight. Likewise, there are many people flying above the magnetic pull of the refrigerator right now, despite early skepticism and ridicule directed at the Weigh Down Workshop[†].

The law of sin (overeating, smoking, alcohol overindulgence, drug overindulgence, materialism, etc.) is somewhat like the law of gravity in that it is real, it is strong, it pulls you down, and it is a force that must be reckoned with. If you have never addressed this compelling force head-on, then you might have some bruises when you begin the process of overcoming. Strongholds are well named. You can ignore the law of gravity and come to an early death. In the same way, you can ignore this law of sin (the magnetic pull to the love of worldly things) and come to an early spiritual death.

Everyone has heard that God, through Jesus, set us free from the law of sin. So why are there so many people still in bondage?

Have you ever thought about how an eagle or a jet airliner can fly? My father loved to fly a single-engine airplane, and the only way we could soar above the clouds was for the right combination of lift and thrust to overcome the forces of load and drag.

Load and drag, respectively, result from gravity and air friction. Lift and thrust are the forward, spread-wing movements. The eagle uses its wings and its muscle power to provide lift and thrust to overcome gravity and friction. In a similar way, an airplane uses its wings and power from its engines. The lift and thrust *we* will discuss are symbolized in the following scripture:

> Those who live according to the sinful nature have their minds set on what that nature desires; but those who live in accordance with the Spirit have their minds set on what the Spirit desires. The mind of sinful man is death, but the mind controlled by the Spirit is life and peace; the sinful mind is hostile to God. It does not submit to God's law, nor can it do so. Those controlled by

the sinful nature cannot please God. (Romans 8:5–8)
Do you see a real key to flying above the gravity of sin or overeating? Focus. Focusing on what God wants. Do not focus on what the flesh or earthly nature wants; get your mind off the food. Every time your mind wanders to food, quickly take it off and ask God to help you focus on Him or His will. Leave the room if you have to. Open the Bible and read God's word. Eating when you are hungry and stopping when you are full is possible when you focus on what God wants. You *will* be successful. And you will fly above the food. This means the gravitational pull of the food will be manageable because your mind is on the will of God. *Focus* is the key, your "lift and thrust." This can be applied to cigarettes, alcohol, antidepressants, diet pills, sexual lusts . . . I can fill up the page with other worldly desires.

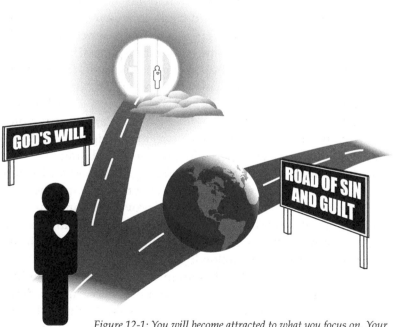

Figure 12-1: You will become attracted to what you focus on. Your footsteps will follow your heart. If you focus on God's will, you will rise above the magnetic pull of the world. If you focus on the world, you will desire it, and that will lead to sin and guilt.

Focusing refers to several things: focusing on the long-term reward and not the short-term desire for food, focusing on what God wants rather than giving in to what the flesh wants, and concentrating on others in place of self. It is like teaching your children to save their money for later, for something that is bigger. We must set our minds on things above. It is just like the scripture that says those who wait in hope upon the Lord will soar on wings like eagles (Isaiah 40:31). Why? Because they are focusing upon the most important and leaving the less important behind.

I love the song that says, "Rise up, O men of God. Have done with lesser things. Give heart, and soul, and mind, and strength to serve the King of Kings."* Do you know how to set your sights on the big things and have nothing to do with the lesser things? This focus that we are talking about is big stuff. In fact, as you get into it, you are going to see that all of this is bigger than you had anticipated. It affects the rest of your day.

Physical exercise is fine, but spend your mind and your strength on this mental exercise. Spend time reading, looking at the right things, praying, listening to Scripture or Weigh Down Workshop† tapes, going to a Weigh Down† class, and helping someone else in class.

The way you fly and finally break away from the pull of the world is to focus on what our heavenly Father wants. Keep your mind centered every day by asking Him, "What do You want, God? Your will, not mine." *Keep your mind off food!*

Getting back on track

Recently, we saw the movie *Hook* starring Robin Williams and Dustin Hoffman. It is a movie about Peter Pan as an adult who has forgotten all about Never-Never Land, Captain Hook, and Tinker Bell. In this version of the story, Peter has even forgotten who he once was, and he has forgotten how to fly. As the children try to help jog his memory, Tinker Bell teaches him to fly again. She tells him to con-

---

* "Rise Up, O Men of God!" Words by William P. Merrill (W. 1911), Music by Aaron Williams (W. 1763).

centrate on happy thoughts. The next thing you know, this grown man is flying as he remembers how to focus on the positive. He can fly because he is concentrating on happy thoughts.

Think on God's way and His long-term rewards and practice, practice, practice. That is the key to flying. A mother eagle teaches her young to fly by pushing them out of the nest. They instinctively hold out their wings. You, too, will have one wing out this week and the next wing out next week.

Many times, the mother eagle will have to swoop down and grab her babies to keep them from falling too far. She puts them back and does it again. They eventually build up coordination to apply enough lift and thrust to overcome the load and the drag. We can help push you out of the nest by encouraging you to focus. It does not hurt. You will be in no pain.

You may need to regroup and restart when you find you are unfocused. One method you may wish to try is fasting. Try not eating for as long as God leads you to. Why empty your body of food? The reason is that emptying out may often help take your body's energy off of the digesting of food and it gives you a focused mind. This extra boost of energy helps you funnel your attention back to your goals: to stop grabbing for food and to wait on God to supply your needs.

Current diet counsel suggests that fasting will damage lean body mass and deprivation will cause you to binge uncontrollably. This is incorrect. Fasting leads to more control. Fasting is all over the Old and the New Testaments as an offering to God. God would not be asking us to damage the body. Fasting has been used for breaking strongholds. The one stronghold that fasting should *not* be used against is anorexia nervosa. The anorexic must not fast anymore, but be obedient to hunger or emptiness by eating every time they sense emptiness.

Remember, fasting is not a goal in the Weigh Down Workshop[†]. It is a means to an end and not an end to itself. Fasting could be used in the beginning of Weigh Down Workshop[†] or when you really have gotten off track.

How does it feel to rise above overeating?

This is how it feels to fly above the food: you could not pay me to overeat. I have absolutely no desire to eat beyond full. In fact, it is almost nauseating to think about overeating. This is the case with other areas in life. Consider stealing, a behavior that arises from worldly greed. Could I pay you right now to go to the mall, steal something from the department store, and bring it back to me? Most people say, with disgust, "No." They are flying above the worldly pull of stealing.

You are going to fly above the pull of food and feel the same way. You will find yourself experiencing strange things. The attraction of food is lessened. You seem to be floating when you can leave food on your plate. The magnetic pull is less when you can actually look up from the food and forget it temporarily. You start realizing that someone else has his face in the food. And, after you finish the meal, you might notice that, for the first time, you did not mind serving others the best and the biggest steak. You did not mind sharing your meal with your children! Halfway through a candy bar, you find you actually can let it go. Amazing! You can wrap it up and put it away. You may not find it in your purse until next week, because you forgot about it. That is flying!

What is happening to you? You have conquered gravity by having the same mindset as Jesus Christ. That is just one of the keys Christ gave us. Look at the rest of this scripture in Romans 8:9–14:

> You, however, are controlled not by the sinful nature but by the Spirit, if the Spirit of God lives in you. And if anyone does not have the Spirit of Christ, he does not belong to Christ. But if Christ is in you, your body is dead because of sin, yet your spirit is alive because of righteousness. And if the Spirit of him who raised Jesus from the dead is living in you, he who raised Christ from the dead will also give life to your mortal bodies through his Spirit, who lives in you.

> Therefore, brothers, we have an obligation —but it is not to the sinful nature, to live according to it. For if you live according to the sinful nature, you will die; but if by the Spirit you put to death the misdeeds of the body, you will live, because those who

are led by the Spirit of God are sons of God.

The Spirit of Christ is not just some vapor or mist. The Spirit of God and Christ that is referred to has deep meaning, and part of that is reflected in the individual's "mindset." In other words, you need to have the same focus as Christ. What was the mindset of Christ? To please the Father and to do His will. That attitude, although just a part of the makeup of the "Spirit of Christ" that is talked about in this passage, is still a part. If that is the case, then you are talking about the power that raised Christ Jesus from the dead. This power will give life to our mortal bodies!

The sun, being much larger than the earth, has a much stronger gravitational pull. We are not conscious of it because we are so close to the earth and so far from the sun. However, if a spaceship were to be launched out of earth's orbit, it would begin moving toward the sun's gravitational pull. The farther it traveled, the less earth's gravity would affect it and the greater the sun's attraction would become.

We want you to pull away from the world and turn your path toward God. As your spaceship draws nearer to God, you will discover that He will draw near to you; He and His ways will become increasingly attractive to you. You will become unable to resist His will because His powerful, magnetic, wonderful force is much, much stronger than the world's pull. You should never want to go back to the world. You will feel like you are floating above the world's lure.

Now, when you mess up and you find that the gravity of sin has pulled your face back down into your plate, or into the refrigerator, or has made you drive your car to the fast food restaurant when you are not hungry, then you need to refocus. Get down on your knees and pray. Ask God to refocus your mind. Just push your restart button; you have one, and you do not have to wait until Monday morning to push it and wait for your next hunger.

Start now. People who wait may never do it. I know about those people who say they are going to start over tomorrow. That means, "I don't want to do it." Why would you start over tomorrow if you *wanted* to do it? Start right now whether you feel like it or not.

Just as sad thoughts brought Peter Pan back down to the ground, preoccupation with your lusts (food, fat grams, exercise, menus, new diets, and planning a binge) will pull you down. Did you fall down? If you did, you focused on your own desires, which are the opposite of God's, while you were being tested.

Do not be deceived; God cannot be mocked. A man reaps what he sows. The one who sows to please his sinful nature, from that nature, will reap destruction; the one who sows to please the Spirit, from the Spirit will reap eternal life. (Galatians 6:7,8)

The purpose of focusing on God

So how much of our mind do we have to give to the Father? That is a good question. We have already started with putting our mind on the Father every time we feel this desire eating or head hunger.

So, we asked you to start thinking about God when your mind wanders or starts lusting after food, which could happen frequently. Dieting has increased your lust for foods over the last few years. Therefore, you might have to get your focus off food and onto God many times a day!

But perhaps that is God's purpose. God has taken something that was occupying our mind and has asked us to transfer that over to Him. This is part of the purpose of the desert. Look at this instructional passage for God's children in Numbers 9:15–23:

On the day the tabernacle, the Tent of the Testimony, was set up, the cloud covered it. From evening till morning the cloud above the tabernacle looked like fire. That is how it continued to be; the cloud covered it, and at night it looked like fire. Whenever the cloud lifted from above the Tent, the Israelites set out; wherever the cloud settled, the Israelites encamped. At the LORD's command the Israelites set out, and at his command they encamped. As long as the cloud stayed over the tabernacle, they remained in camp. When the cloud remained over the tabernacle a long time, the Israelites obeyed the LORD's order and did not set out. Sometimes the cloud was over the tabernacle only a few days; at the LORD's command they would encamp, and then at his command they would set out. Sometimes the cloud stayed only from evening till morning, and when it lifted in the morning, they set out. Whether by day or by night, whenever the cloud

lifted, they set out. Whether the cloud stayed over the tabernacle
for two days or a month or a year, the Israelites would remain in
camp and not set out; but when it lifted, they would set out. At
the LORD's command they encamped, and at the LORD's command they set out. They obeyed the LORD's order, in accordance
with his command through Moses.

Think about this assignment if you start to feel sorry that you have
to look to God to know when you are hungry and look to God to
know when you are full. The Israelites had to look up all day and
night. If it was in the middle of the night, they had to pack their
tents, put out the fires, gather the children and pets, and take off.
Sometimes, just after they had unpacked their belongings, set up
the tent, and had a good pot of manna boiling, God lifted the cloud,
and they had to pack everything up and take off again. Let us stop
complaining about a red light and green light with food. All you
will have to pack up is a carryout of food! Have you noticed that it
takes your whole mind to get the red light and green light with hunger and fullness down correctly? God wants it all. But when we make
Him the master of our minds, we are free from the pull of food.
Sounds good to me! Since we are going to be a slave to one or the
other, I choose God!

Conclusion

We need to stay focused on what the Spirit of God wants.

Finally, brothers, whatever is true, whatever is noble, whatever
is right, whatever is pure, whatever is lovely, whatever is admi-
rable, if anything is excellent or praiseworthy, *think* about such
things. (Philippians 4:8)

Just as there were early skeptics who thought pioneer aviators could
not overcome Earth's gravity, skeptics today do not believe that you
can overcome sin. Those skeptics will tell you that your efforts are
getting you nowhere, too. They will tell you that you are wasting
your time. They will tell you that you are crazy—you cannot reach
your goal without depending on fat grams and exercise as your savior. They will cry out, "So where is your God that is supposed to
rescue you? Maybe He cannot hear you." Your enemies will watch

you fly above the food for a few days, hoping to see you crash. They love to distract you and they beg you to fixate on fat grams instead of heavenly things. Skeptics are inside and outside the church building. Some of them are living with you. They say once an alcoholic, always an alcoholic; or once you become obese, you will just have to watch it for the rest of your life. They have never seen a rocket orbit around the earth beyond the pull of the world. But I would ask them whether they have read or heard of 1 Peter 4:1,2:

> Therefore, since Christ suffered in his body, arm yourselves also with the same attitude, because he who has suffered in his body is done with sin. As a result, he does not live the rest of his earthly life for evil human desires, but rather for the will of God.

Is that not about the most exciting thing you have ever read? Not only have I experienced it, but I have witnessed it firsthand in these small group sessions; and I have received truckloads of letters, not to mention thousands of phone calls. You do not have to listen to that voice again. You can *fly*, and you can eventually pull far enough away from the world (food) to escape its pull. Skeptics have never flown high enough to break loose of its gravity and soar freely. I have broken free of the refrigerator's pull, and it no longer exerts a gravitational pull on me.

Do not concentrate on the enemy or enemies. That is part of the Weigh Down Workshop[†] homework God gives us. We will be like the pioneer pilots who, against all odds, reached their goals by setting their minds on what was not seen rather than what was seen— their skeptics and the early, inevitable failures. You do the same.

> Therefore we do not lose heart. Though outwardly we are wasting away, yet inwardly we are being renewed day by day. For our light and momentary troubles are achieving for us an eternal glory that far outweighs them all. So we fix our eyes not on what is seen, but on what is unseen. For what is seen is temporary, but what is unseen is eternal. (2 Corinthians 4:16–18)

Remember, a great way to put our mind on the Father is to go to the Word of God. Carry your Bible around with you. Take it on the subway. Leave a copy at your desk at work. You will start the transferring process from food to God's word and get to the point that you can say as Job did, "I have treasured the words of his mouth more than my daily bread" (Job 23:12b).

Another great way is just to talk to God. Pray that you will not be led into temptation, but that you will be delivered from the evil desire. Jesus taught us to pray for that. So what if you have to pray it twenty times a day!?

Here is Jesus's prayer that I paraphrased from Matthew 6:9–13, and Luke 11:2–4:

Dear Heavenly Father:

Hallowed be your name. (How awesome and above all you are.)

Your kingdom come. (We pray that Your ideas, government, justice, and ways to live come and replace this worldly way of life because Your kingdom is perfect.)

Give us this day our daily bread. (Give us this day the portion we need.)

Lead us not into temptation. (Guide us out of tempting situations.)

And deliver us from the evil one.

For yours is the kingdom, the power, and the glory forever. (After all, You are It. And you are everything. You are all-powerful. You are who we worship, admire, and adore.)

Amen.

We started this book with the passage from Colossians that states that man-made rules have no value in restraining sensual indulgence. The next sentence tells you what does have value in restraining sensual indulgence. Look at this missing key to rising above the captivation of the kitchen:

Since then, you have been raised with Christ, set your hearts on things above where Christ is seated at the right hand of God. Set your *minds* on things above, not on earthly things. For you died, and your life is now hidden, with Christ in God. (Colossians 3:1–3)

God wants your mind. When I gave Him my mind, He cleaned it up and made it pure, and He placed inside it more understanding than I had ever had before. He wants your *mind*, too. *Give it to Him*, for you will get much in return.

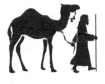

THE DESERT OF TESTING

Love the Lord with all of your heart . . .

L et us now explore the Desert of Testing. This desert is an opportunity—not a curse—to learn much about the Father and yourself. Continuing with the scripture that has been entitled the "Greatest Commandment" (Mark 12:28–34) . . .

One of the teachers of the law came and heard them debating. Noticing that Jesus had given them a good answer, he asked him, "Of all the commandments, which is the most important?"

"The most important one," answered Jesus, "is this: 'Hear, O Israel, the Lord our God, the Lord is one. Love the Lord your God with all your heart and with all your soul and with all your mind and with all your strength.' The second is this: 'Love your neighbor as yourself.' There is no commandment greater than these."

"Well said, teacher," the man replied. "You are right in saying that God is one and there is no other but him. To love him with all your heart, with all your understanding and with all your strength, and to love your neighbor as yourself is more important than all burnt offerings and sacrifices."

When Jesus saw that he had answered wisely, he said to him,

"You are not far from the kingdom of God." And from then on
no one dared ask him any more questions.

Why did Jesus say, "You are not far from the kingdom of heaven?"
Why could He not just have said, "You hit the nail on the head; you
understand it and you have got it," to the man who answered wisely?
Because just having the *knowledge* of what God is looking for is not
enough.

The journey has to start in the mind, as we discussed in the last
chapter. But you could have the knowledge of God and not have a
heart for Him at all. Love God with *all* your heart, the scripture says.
Your first question might be: "What is your heart?"

The best way to describe *loving with your heart* is to liken it to the
love we have for another person. If you have ever had a crush on
someone, then you know how this feels. You feel your emotions rise
and your pulse rate goes up. You would know if your lover entered
the room even if you did not see him or her, for your senses are alert
to the voice and presence of the one you love. Your mind thinks
about your lover every spare moment, including times that it should
be concentrating on the job at hand. You clean up and dress for your
lover. You look for opportunities to be in his or her presence. You
look forward to your times alone. You would do anything for this
person and find it no problem; providing aid would be a pleasure.
Being separated brings sadness. That is your heart. It is an emotional entity. It is passion and feeling.

Let me give you one of my sample days, strictly for reasons of
comparison, to show you how it looks to have a heart for God.

Sample day of a passionate heart

It has not always been this way, but let me start with the beginning
of the day. I have not set an alarm clock in many years. God wakes
me up. Do you believe that? Even if I need a special, out-of-the-
routine time early in the morning, I just make my special request to
my Heavenly Father. Sure enough, God wakes me up at just the
right time. Yes, He accomplishes this without using an obnoxious
alarm clock buzzer that would send painful adrenaline out into my
stomach. With gentle creativity, He chooses a variety of waking

methods. Fifteen years ago, I gave my eating signal over to God; now I have given my wake-up signal over to Him as well. If I awaken in the night, I talk to God; and as He wakes me in the morning, I look out the window for Him and sometimes wink at Him. I always look to see what kind of day He has made. I love them all—rainy, cold, hot . . . they are all awesome.

The rest of the day follows suit. The Bible says to "pray without ceasing." Therefore, every hour is spent talking to Him, looking for His opinion, asking Him to rule my day, asking Him to find my keys, thanking Him for something that just happened, coming to Him for comfort from pain in the heart, and looking to Him for His attention or approval and leading any way I can get it. After all, He is the CEO of this world. I ask Him for help with all my daily work.

When I find myself alone in a room or the entire house, I sing to Him my made-up, on-the-spot songs of adoration for His great personality, His mighty hand of justice, and His protection for the righteous. I also listen to music, and now I interpret most love songs as His singing to us, since love and romance were all His own idea. I praise Him for His great ideas. For example, what great ideas are twenty-four-hour days, sleep, and snuggling up in the covers with my pillow over my head while I talk to Him. After all, He is the one who made covers and pillows and the snuggly feeling. I praise Him for humor, for incredibly *moving* music that He inspires, for happy-go-lucky children and puppy dogs, for smiling faces, and for the genius of different types of food.

I praise Him for making weather different every single day so that the land, the clouds, and the sky change colors. I praise Him for putting love and peace in our hearts so there are not only smiles on our faces but also empathy for others in our hearts. The great idea list is endless. Do I sound childlike? *Good!*

What a genius and yet a powerful King we have an opportunity to serve! He opens my eyes daily to new information from His Word or from life that confirms He is the source of everything. So I love Him as a teacher, a comforter, a constant companion, a trustworthy leader, a husband/defender when I am slandered or falsely accused, an hour-by-hour boss, the source of life, and the love of my life to whom I can confidently give my love and passion.

It means everything to have His love returned to me. I long to see His face. I have no doubt that I will know Him, and my heart will pound like that of a schoolgirl with a crush, for it does so even now! It is easy to love others with all this love that I have in my heart. I can return love even to others who hurt me because I *know* He loves me. Others might hurt me, but God's opinion is so much higher on my list that it does not matter so much anymore what others may do. 1 Peter 1:8 describes my feelings:

> Though you have not seen Him, you love Him; and even though you do not see Him now, you believe in Him and are filled with an inexpressible and glorious joy.

When I think about how involved He is in my life, I sometimes want to cry. Obviously, there are hurting and sad times too, but even in the low points, my heart always runs to the Father and finds peace only in Him.

This is the end of my sample day.

As you can see, it is not a good idea to get me started because I can't quit! I really cannot be silent about God. I am moved just thinking about Him.

Seeing the passion

Now, I am aware that sounds a lot like *emotional religion*. But reason with me for a minute. There are many people out there who say that God does not want "emotional religion." And there are others who say they are burnt out in life. These people supposedly do not have this kind of emotion to give God, so they could not give it even if they wanted to.

Wrong! God made our hearts, and you do have one. In fact, we all have the same size heart, and we all have one hundred percent of a heart—but some people have given pieces of their heart to other things. These pieces of their heart are so scattered about that they do not have the energy to be passionate about any single thing!

Many people have idols in their lives and are not even aware of what they are giving their devotion and energy to. There is only one way to find out if something is an idol in your life: let it be taken away. Then, if you really mourn for it, you know that your heart has been given over to an idol. For example, if God took away your food, how would you react? It could be that you have the same diagnosis as these people that Paul wrote about in Philippians 3:18,19: "For, as I have often told you before and now say again even with tears, many live as enemies of the cross of Christ. Their destiny is destruction, their god is their stomach, and their glory is in their shame. Their mind is on earthly things."

There is nothing wrong with any of these things listed below—it is your heart. God weighs the *motives* of the heart. If you worship something else, you will feel drained, lethargic, worn-out, and emo-

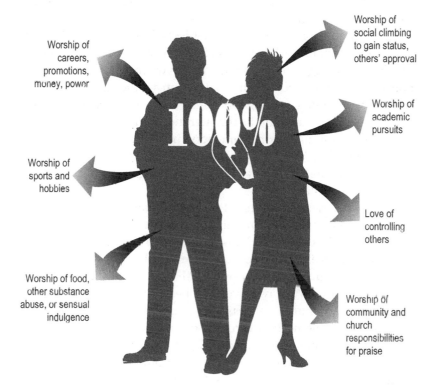

Figure 13-1: Each of us chooses where and how to invest one hundred percent of our heart, passion, and devotion. Unless we give them all to God, we tend to divide them among many activities and causes, dissipating ourselves to the point that we have no great passion for any particular one of them. Passion given to the world drains you; passion given to God is given back to you by God, and you are energized.

tionless. You will not have energy to love your spouse, children, or friends. You will feel empty because you never get what you are after. God will not let your false god give you what you are looking for. None of them will *fill* you up.

However, if you throw yourself into worshipping God, then He will guide you to do things. This will not be draining, but rewarding. The externals may look the same, but the product and the fruit produced by your activities will be very different: one you directed, one He directed. Your energy level will rise. Your joy will be great!

People have put their hearts into football and basketball, computers and cars, clothes and social climbing, chocolate and desserts, children and careers. Name it, and it can be an idol.

You may still argue that you do not feel all that emotional toward anything, but think with me again. If I were to lock you up in a room that had no refrigerator or pantry in it, you might start off asking politely for some food. A while later, you would ask a little more forcefully. As time goes on, you might resort to begging and bribing. Eventually you would be threatening, yelling and screaming at me to let you out or to bring some food in. Some people might even kill for food. Don't tell me you haven't broken in a buffet line or jumped out of the car to get ahead of the next group of people going into the same restaurant.

So, you tell me: is that kind of person *emotional* about their food? Is that passion or what? I have known of grown men who stole money from their children's piggy banks in order to sneak away and feed their own obsessive greed for food. We may have chosen to devote our heart to food. Put another way, we have a "crush" on food; food is our stronghold. We have given our heart to food.

I have sat in church on a Sunday evening and watched people listlessly drag themselves through the motions of their worship. These are the same people who will put on one blue shoe and one white one, wave a blue and white pom-pom, and apply blue and white paint on their faces to root for their favorite college teams. They jump up after the worship service (sad name for what took place) and rush to basketball games. They may know the name of every player and every statistic, and once at the game, they scream, yell, and jump up and down for the players. But can these same people tell you much about the heavenly team or any of its star players—Jesus, Abraham, and David? So we do have a heart, and we do know how to worship something . . . it may just be misplaced.

If you have a crush on God and think it may go away and be replaced by a "more mature," emotionless love, think again. Your love for food grows more and more. Statistics show us that people in developed countries are getting larger and larger and more and more passionate for their food. Likewise, my love for God has grown more and more. I can't get Him out of my heart and mind. It is passion, and that is how God wants it. It is either growing for one and departing from the other, or vice versa. "No one can serve two masters" (Matthew 6:24). Why? Because you only have one heart. It is made to be devoted. It will *not* be devoted to two things. It cannot be. It is not possible.

So how do you transfer your passion?

There are two things you need to know to help with this realignment. Number one is to open your eyes to what a life-sucking leech the god of food is and what a life-replenisher is the one true God. Number two, practically speaking, is a crash course on "how to fall in love" with God.

Exposing the false god

Let us start by exposing this master, this friend called food. Just how good of a friend has excessive food been to us? (Note: Our daily allotted food is not a false god—we are referring to excessive food.)

Does overeating help our finances? No, it robs us. It is expensive to keep eating extra calories every day. Diet programs have emptied our savings accounts as well. Does it help us with our clothing? No, we tend to find less and less to wear as we find ourselves obeying food more and more. Does it help us with our self-esteem? No, the more the excessive food is a friend to us, the more it gathers on our hips and in other locations of the body, and the more our self-esteem drops. Does it help us with our relationships? No, it seems to put a wedge between us and our families or spouses.

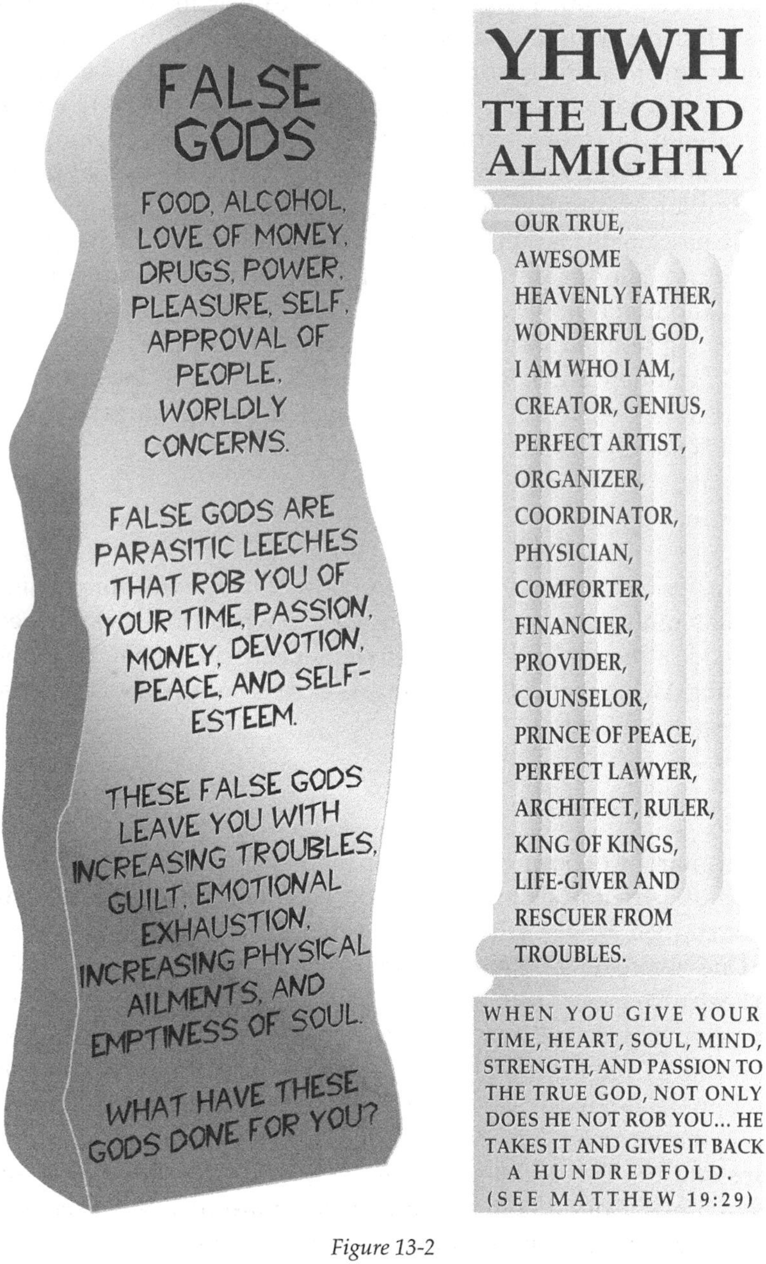

FALSE GODS

FOOD, ALCOHOL, LOVE OF MONEY, DRUGS, POWER, PLEASURE, SELF, APPROVAL OF PEOPLE, WORLDLY CONCERNS.

FALSE GODS ARE PARASITIC LEECHES THAT ROB YOU OF YOUR TIME, PASSION, MONEY, DEVOTION, PEACE, AND SELF-ESTEEM.

THESE FALSE GODS LEAVE YOU WITH INCREASING TROUBLES, GUILT, EMOTIONAL EXHAUSTION, INCREASING PHYSICAL AILMENTS, AND EMPTINESS OF SOUL.

WHAT HAVE THESE GODS DONE FOR YOU?

YHWH
THE LORD ALMIGHTY

OUR TRUE, AWESOME HEAVENLY FATHER, WONDERFUL GOD, I AM WHO I AM, CREATOR, GENIUS, PERFECT ARTIST, ORGANIZER, COORDINATOR, PHYSICIAN, COMFORTER, FINANCIER, PROVIDER, COUNSELOR, PRINCE OF PEACE, PERFECT LAWYER, ARCHITECT, RULER, KING OF KINGS, LIFE-GIVER AND RESCUER FROM TROUBLES.

WHEN YOU GIVE YOUR TIME, HEART, SOUL, MIND, STRENGTH, AND PASSION TO THE TRUE GOD, NOT ONLY DOES HE NOT ROB YOU... HE TAKES IT AND GIVES IT BACK A HUNDREDFOLD. (SEE MATTHEW 19:29)

Figure 13-2

Extra food turns out to be a false friend and a parasitic leech that robs us of our time, passion, money, devotion, peace, and self-esteem. It is a false master, a false friend, or a false god that leaves us with increasing troubles, guilt, emotional deprivation, and physical ailments.

Look at the irony. We have been running to the refrigerator for comfort. In Figure 13-2, there is a statue of a false god and a column that represents our true God. We need to evaluate ourselves this week and every week from here on: what percentage of time have we been running to God and what percentage have we been running to the refrigerator or any false god? Time is a great indicator of what we give our heart to.

As has already been pointed out, God has it all and is very generous to hearts that love Him. You may not really believe He is there and is that personal, but what if He is, and you have just missed it?! It is time to give Him a try, if you have not already. If you run to Him for everything, you will be rewarded with great dividends or jewels. This way you can prove that He exists and rewards those who diligently seek Him. "And without faith it is impossible to please God, because anyone who comes to him must believe that he exists and that he rewards those who earnestly seek him" (Hebrews 11:6). Running to God for comfort and solutions makes sense. Do you need a counselor? He knows all truth, and His word is a light unto your path. Do you need a friend? He is the God of all comfort. Are you low in money, need your roof fixed or your car repaired? I have seen some pretty incredible things happen through prayer. Are you looking for excitement? His kingdom is dynamic. There is nothing that He cannot do. He sometimes uses people to solve the problem, and sometimes He does not. He is creative, and you will know it is from Him.

Crash course on how to fall in love

Now for the crash course on how to fall in love. Well, how did we fall in love with food?

What happened was that our hearts became enslaved to food by obeying the food. When the potato chips called our name from the pantry and said, "Hey, come eat me," we found ourselves listening and obeying. When we drove down the street and the #3 combo from the fast food restaurant called our name, we found ourselves obeying by pulling into the drive-through. When we thought about a great steak dinner, we felt our emotions rise. Our pulse rate went up. Our senses were alert to the voice and presence of food (popcorn popping, steak sizzling, corn boiling, and candy wrappers opening). Our mind thought about recipes and dinners every spare moment, including times when it should have been concentrating on the job at hand. We found ourselves dressing for eating occasions, preferring elastic outfits with no belts! We looked for opportunities to be in the food's presence. We looked forward to times alone for a binge. We found ourselves showing outwardly recognizable emotions when we thought about dessert or chips and dip. We would do anything to get to food and find it no problem. Cooking something is always a pleasure. Being separated from food brings sadness. Slowly but surely, this describes the state of your heart. Your heart is an emotional, feeling entity. Does all this sound parallel to the crush I described earlier?

We love the master that we obey. And we obey the master we love. We cannot love both God and food. Either we will hate the one and love the other or we will love the one and hate the other. Do not kid yourself—you cannot be in love with God if you are in love with food! And do not expect God to believe that you are in love with Him at the same time you are in love with food. He knows better.

Even though the thought and smell of food is what got me out of the bed in the morning years ago—now all my senses are given over to God. I dress for Him. I can sense (even though I do not see Him) when He is near. I can kind of tell when He is calling me to read His word. All senses are alive for Him. One workshop participant told me that she does not call it coincidence anymore, but "God-incidence!"

Notice that there is nothing inherently wrong with alcohol, tobacco, food, credit cards, tranquilizers, and sexual desire. What is wrong is with our heart. Tearing up the credit card is not going to keep our heart from materialism. Making the food have less fat is not going to make our heart less greedy for food. Locking someone up in a detoxification center to bring them down off alcohol or substance abuse is not going to fix their heart.

We fell in love with the food by giving it our heart, soul, mind, and strength, which is included in this one behavior called obedience. We obeyed it. It called us from the bed in the morning, and we used our strength to prepare it. We also used our strength to force more of it down into the body than the body called for. We gave it our mind all day long by looking through recipe books and discussing the latest diets with our friends, asking, "What do you get to eat on your diet?" We lusted after the foods that were on the menu, and we gave our hearts to the 10 o'clock binge.

To convert this love for the refrigerator—we need to obey God. Every time we obey God with regard to food or with anything He is putting on our heart to work on, we will fall more in love with Him. Partly, this is because "He rewards those who earnestly seek him" (Hebrews 11:6). (Note: we are to earnestly [with a true heart] seek Him—not His money or His power—but Him.) And part of the reason we fall in love through obedience, or keeping His commands, is that He answers the prayers of those who obey Him. John 14:14 says, "You may ask me for anything in my name, and I will do it."

Consider again Deuteronomy 8:2: "Remember how the LORD your God led you all the way in the desert these forty years, to humble you and to test you in order to know what was in your heart, *whether or not you would keep his commands.*" From the context of this passage, it looks like obedience is a big factor in knowing what is truly in our hearts. This assumption is backed up by the words spoken by Jesus. He said it first one way and then He would turn it around and say it another. You would think that He was making sure that we got the message while He was down on earth. Take a look:

"If you love me, you will obey what I command." (John 14:15)

"Whoever has my commands and obeys them, he is the one who loves me. He who loves me will be loved by my Father, and I too will love him and show myself to him." (John 14:21)

"If anyone loves me, he will obey my teaching. My Father will love him, and we will come to him and make our home

with him. He who does not love me will not obey my teaching."
(John 14:23,24a)
    "As the Father has loved me, so have I loved you. Now remain in my love. If you obey my commands, you will remain in my love, just as I have obeyed my Father's commands and remain in his love. I have told you this so that my joy may be in you and that your joy may be complete." (John 15:9–11)
    We know that we have come to know him if we obey his commands. The man who says, "I know him," but does not do what he commands is a liar, and the truth is not in him. But if anyone obeys his word, God's love is truly made complete in him. This is how we know we are in him: Whoever claims to live in him must walk as Jesus did. (1 John 2:3–6)
So obedience is certainly one major—if not *the* major—way to measure the love in our heart for God and to make love for God grow in our heart. After all, it is what we use for knowing if our children love us, trust us, and respect us. Obedience is also the acid test for employers to know the hearts of employees. Patronizing obedience and false love are always easily detected.

Obedience is not the destination of our desert journey. Rather, it is the means to the end: the love of God.

    The obedience that God calls for is obedience to His commands. So what are His commands? First, to love Him with all our heart. Second, to love our neighbor as ourselves. Does this sound like we are going in circles? It kind of does to me. It looks as if the genuine article—the heart that truly does love God—will, at the same time, be obedient by loving God and others. Love and obedience walk hand in hand. They feed each other so that your love for God and other people grows more and more.

    For my own Desert of Testing, it was only because I loved Him that I obeyed Him in the beginning. The beginning was very hard, and it brought many tears and much pain to rip the idols out of my life. Once I had obeyed Him, I loved, trusted, and respected His commands even more and loved the idols less. This made it easier the next time. With each bite of food you push away out of pure obedience to God, the more you will love Him. The next sacrifice will be easier as you see more and more rewards coming from the Father. Love is inevitable as you obey Him. The love for food will disappear—salvation! Salvation from your old master (food) and permission to give yourself to God.

From reading the Old Testament, you notice that the Israelites went in and out of worship to idols. As a result, God would then enslave them to the wicked surrounding countries. After a burdensome and painful enslavement, they would repent and turn their hearts back to the Father, and He would free them. So obedience and freedom go together, as do disobedience and slavery. That is true with you and food. Disobedience and miserable dieting go hand in hand. Obedience to God using hunger and fullness (or a lack of greed for food), as well as freedom to eat what you want, also go hand in hand. Obedience is not the destination of our desert journey. Rather, it is the means to the end: *the love of God.*

The golden calf

As you go through the journey in the desert, you may see several things about your heart that had not occurred to you before. Just what you are giving your heart to is something only God knows. This hot desert acts as an X-ray machine, revealing the inner workings of the heart.

So we find we have been bowing down to the refrigerator. The New Testament talks about greed as idolatry. "Put to death, therefore, whatever belongs to your earthly nature: sexual immorality, impurity, lust, evil desires and greed, which is idolatry" (Colossians 3:5). Why is greed idolatry? Greed is idolatry in that we are trying to get things for ourselves. We do not believe in our hearts that there is a loving God who will meet all of our needs, and we certainly do not believe that He satisfies our wants. What if God does not have good taste in foods or material possessions? Who would want to include God on a shopping spree? He may not let us have upscale, brand-name shoes.

And what do we know of God's timing? Perhaps His watch is

broken or He is helping people on the other side of the world. We do not want to bother Him with details. We may think, "To get in good with God, it will be best not to bother Him until we need the big stuff, right?" Wrong!

That thinking led the Israelites to create their own false god. Remember the story we told earlier about the golden calf? The Israelites wanted to get out of the desert fast. Moses had ascended a mountain to receive God's laws on stone tablets.

When the people saw that Moses was so long in coming down from the mountain, they gathered around Aaron and said, "Come, make us gods who will go before us . . . .

So all the people took off their earrings and brought them to Aaron. He took what they handed him and made it into an idol cast in the shape of a calf . . . . (Exodus 32:1a,3–4a)

When considerable time had passed and the Israelites did not see Moses coming back—so as not to bother God and in case His watch was broken—they made a golden calf to help speed things up. Of course, Israel's worship of the golden calf made God angry. Moses, himself angry, threw down the tablets God had made, breaking them. The Israelites had to wait *another* forty days for Moses as he replaced them.

We are no different from the Israelites. We, too, are willing to give up our jewelry to keep paying for our false gods—false helpers. We carve out an exercise/diet pill regimen to speed up our journey because we do not want to eat less food. We say, "Don't tell Gwen, but let's mix Weigh Down† with diet pills to get us out of this desert faster." You will only stay in the desert longer because your heart does not want to eat less food.

Many will attempt mixing diuretics with Weigh Down Workshop†. This may give them a false sense of security, but they should realize that diuretics could damage their kidneys.

We hope false gods will save us, but they will get us nowhere. Can false gods take away our desire to overeat? They cannot. Truth bears out that our false gods sabotage us rather than save us! Trying to worship God and food at the same time will not work.

The Matthew 19:29 principle

We cannot run to false gods to get us out of our pain, and we cannot save ourselves by building golden calves in the form of diet pills, suction surgery, diet programs, hospital liquid diets, and fat farms. We need to give our heart, our soul, our mind, and our strength to obeying God rather than food. We need to develop this relationship with God the Father through Jesus Christ. That is the only way we can come to trust that He truly is the One who can rescue us from our troubles. Then, the next thing we know, we are falling in love with Him. We can forget our old love called food. When we give our heart to Him, the true God, He does not rob us of anything. In fact, He takes our heart, our soul, our mind, and our strength and multiplies them a hundred times and gives them back to us. Just as the false god robs you, the true God gives back great dividends. You give Him the rest of your sandwich; He gives you back the next smaller dress or pants size, along with many other jewels. He is a multibillionaire!

You cannot out-give the one true God. Let me offer you just a few personal examples. As I learned to be directed by Him in little ways, I eventually decided that it was God who is waking me in the night. It took a long time before I made the connection. Then, to be sure, I asked God to make it clear to me. I asked, "If it is You, O Lord, wanting me to get up to read Your Word or to talk to You (pray), then could You wake me with two things at once? For example, Lord, could You wake me having to go to the bathroom *and* blow my nose, or could you combine the moon shining in my eyes and Puss 'n' Boots, our cat, rattling a bowl in the kitchen?"

You see, getting out of bed in the

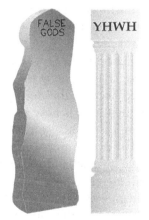

FALSE GODS   YHWH

"And everyone who has left houses or brothers or sisters or father or mother or children or fields for my sake will receive a hundred times as much and will inherit eternal life." (Matthew 19:29)

middle of the night is painful to me. So just as you want to be sure that He really wants you to give the second half of your lunch, I wanted to be sure that He wanted my middle-of-the-night sleep. That is like asking for the heart of the watermelon or the icing on the cake. Believe me, I would only get up in the middle of the night for the one true God—not just any god! So, God would send two things to wake me. For example, one night I got really cold, and at the same time, a portable phone low-battery indicator started beeping. Another night, just after I finished typing a speech I would be taping in the studio the next day, I reasoned with Him to let me sleep, saying that the sleep would help me with the studio talk. Five minutes later, the Christmas tree fell over. It did not take two things that night. I told Him that I did not think that was very funny! (But actually, it was very funny and I knew it!) That night, I rewrote the entire speech for the taping, and it turned out much better than before!

Most nights He would take me to some thrilling new scripture in the Bible or just get me up to see the full moon that He made. Oh, the fun I have had (and still have) with the Father at unknown hours in the morning or during the day. I always did, and still do, keep my heating pad and Bible in my "spot" that I always use for my wintery night rendezvous with God. But since I began to give Him some of my precious sleep time, He has always put me back into a deep sleep and awakened me just in time the next morning. I am never tired because the God of sleep gives it back in a concentrated form. (I guess that is how He does it . . . I really don't know how He accomplishes this—all I know is that it happens.)

Other examples are that I tried giving Him my money, and He gave me back more. Then I gave up my house to help our finances, and He gave me a larger one. He is a God of endless resources. He can give or do anything He pleases. You cannot out-give the Father. I know that the rain falls on the just and the unjust. But it just so happens that it pleases Him to give to those who have a heart for Him. And I am eternally, gratefully in love with Jesus for making the path to the Father clear and available.

I could never have made it this far without Him. He guides me and counsels me. He leads me away from trouble and into pleasant situations. Greed is idolatry; we feel that we need to satisfy our needs ourselves, so we make ourselves the god. How exhausting! We need to believe in God. We need to taste and see that He is good. "Test me in this," says the Lord Almighty, "and see if I will not throw open the floodgates of heaven and pour out so much blessing that you will not have room enough for it." (Malachi 3:10b)

The greatest of these is love

It is time that we wake up and see that being our own god has gotten us nowhere and that bowing down to the world has robbed us blind. Second-rate gods are worthless. We ought to be thankful that God is crazy about us and willing to have us. It is called *grace*.

And God spoke all these words:

"I am the LORD your God, who brought you out of Egypt, out of the land of slavery. "You shall have no other gods before me. "You shall not make for yourself an idol in the form of anything in heaven above or on the earth beneath or in the waters below. You shall not bow down to them or worship them; for I, the LORD your God, am a jealous God, punishing the children for the sin of the fathers to the third and fourth generation of those who hate me, but showing love to a thousand generations of those who love me and keep my commandments." (Exodus 20:1–6)

Having faith in God is great; having hope in God is good; but the greatest of these is being in love with God.

This is a cry from God's heart of "I have made you and I have taken care of you, and I have delivered you. Be in love with and devoted to me only."

It is better to be emptied out in the desert and be with our Great God than to be indulged in the world without God. Plus, those who hang in there through the desert will get to the Promised Land. I cannot wait to tell you about that!

The heart is a tricky thing. You cannot look at the outside or the environment of people to see what is in their hearts. You could have two people eating rich chocolate cake, and one could be sinning and the other not. How is that? One's heart could be committing adultery, and the other's heart be wholeheartedly in love with God—enjoying His bounty, but with a heart *detached* from it.

King David worshipped all the time; his heart loved everything about God. "Oh, how I love your law [your ideas, etc.]! I meditate on it all day long" (Psalm 119:97). Jesus was in love with God, and He said, " '. . . but the world *must* learn that I *love* the Father and that I do exactly what my Father has commanded me . . .' " (John 14:31).

So, the Desert of Testing has been worthwhile to see if there is love in our hearts for God.

Jesus' life defined love. The Apostle Paul loved Jesus and God the Father. It was his very life. Paul teaches us what love means in 1 Corinthians 13:

If I speak in the tongues of men and of angels, but have not love, I am only a resounding gong or a clanging cymbal. If I have the gift of prophecy and can fathom all mysteries and all knowledge, and if I have a faith that can move mountains, but have not love, I am nothing. If I give all I possess to the poor and surrender my body to the flames, but have not love, I gain nothing.

Love is patient, love is kind. It does not envy, it does not boast, it is not proud. It is not rude, it is not self-seeking, it is not easily angered, it keeps no record of wrongs. Love does not delight in evil but rejoices with the truth. It always protects, always trusts, always hopes, always perseveres.

Love never fails. But where there are prophecies, they will cease; where there are tongues, they will be stilled; where there is knowledge, it will pass away. For we know in part and we prophesy in part, but when perfection comes, the imperfect disappears. When I was a child, I talked like a child, I thought like a child, I reasoned like a child. When I became a man, I put childish ways behind me. Now we see but a poor reflection as in a mirror; then we shall see face to face. Now I know in part; then I shall know fully, even as I am fully known.

And now these three remain: faith, hope and love. But the greatest of these is love.

This passage tells me we could give all our possessions and money, give our body to be burned, and be the greatest orator or singer of the century for God; but if we are not in love with God, we are nothing and we gain nothing! When you fall in love with God, you will no longer need all these tutors and professors (tongues and prophecies), because you will have graduated and found the end, *love of God*. Having faith in God is great; having hope in God is good; but the greatest of these is *being in love with God*. And that is the heart of the matter.

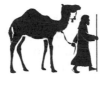

STAY AWAKE

Love the Lord with all of your strength . . .

The Apostle Paul called us many times to be "self-controlled and alert." I have heard people off and on over the last few years say something along these lines: "Well, I think my over-eating is a spiritual problem." I would wonder, "What are they really saying? Are they saying they are spiritually inadequate? Are they saying there are worldly problems (like car trouble) and that weight control is in the realm of the spiritual?" At first, I was not sure what they meant. But I am sure that repenting and turning from our old ways, giving up our will, acknowledging God's way to eat is the right way, resisting temptation by being obedient, and continuing to resist every hour of the day until we are flying above the pull of food are, indeed, spiritual battles. It is tiring enough just talking about this, much less living it!

War has been declared

Your weight is not a spiritual *problem* or *condition*, in the sense of an ailment or affliction that needs a rubdown or heavy dose of a wonder drug. Rather, it is spiritual *warfare* in which you are a soldier. If anything is a problem, it is that bombs are dropping and bullets are flying all around you, but you are not aware of them. You may not even know that you are at war. If you are in this category, no wonder you are getting more and more out of control. You cannot be winning battles if you do not know that a war has been declared.

Knowing and loving God are going to require your strength. Paul described it many times as a "race," and you are straining to get to the finish line. Sometimes what is happening to you is just another pop quiz. But approaching food today without understanding the dynamics of what we are talking about is like taking a college class and spending your time daydreaming or taking naps. The next thing you know, all the students around you are turning in their exam papers, while you did not even know there was an exam! Failing the test is inevitable.

It would be so much simpler, we think, if God could just warn us: "My dear children, you are going to be tested today by Satan, and lured and enticed by your own flesh at 1:15 this afternoon with chocolate cheesecake—and I want you to stop when you are full and wrap up the rest of it. Now get yourself ready for 1:15 today." Too bad it does not work that way. I would have passed many more college pop quizzes if I had known exactly what the test was about and when it would be given. As it was, I had to *stay awake*. I had to stay alert so as to be ready when the professor decided to give me an exam.

I feel sure I could win many more spiritual wars if I knew when to put on my battle armor, where the battle was, who the opponent was, and how to defeat him or it. I would be ready for all those pop quizzes. However, God does not work this way because God wants us always to be battle-ready. He wants us to be focused on Him at all times. If I had to say there was one purpose for the Weigh Down Workshop^{t} and this battle that you are going through with weight, it is that He wants you to keep your eyes fixed on Him at *all* times. If He calls you in the middle of the night, you must answer your General. He will have unannounced pop quizzes to keep your eyes turned upward.

Since we do not know who, what, when, where, and how, the only effective plan is to stay on guard at all times. I have often thought that it is the battle-ready believers who are the most "with it," the most alert, "on top of it" kind of people.

The battlefield

Now let us take a look at this battle or race that we are in. What we are to fight and resist are Satan's lies and our own fleshly desires and temptations to eat more food than the body is calling for (greed). Paul described the location of this battle in Romans 7:21–23 when he said,

> So I find this law at work: When I want to do good, evil is right there with me. For in my inner being I delight in God's law; but I see another law at work in the members of my body, waging war against the law of my *mind* and making me a prisoner of the law of sin at work within my members.

Paul went on to say that the Holy Spirit of Christ sets us free from the law of sin and death. But rest assured that we must constantly battle to submit our wills and train our minds to stay focused on what the law of Christ is; and we must put to death our earthly desires.

So we know where the battle is—it is in the mind and heart. And we have some knowledge of what we are up against in this war—our own fleshly desire or will. We know we will win the war if we stay focused on the Spirit of Jesus Christ and on the will of God. This means we spend our energy getting our minds off our earthly wants as Paul described in Colossians 3:5a: "Put to death, therefore, whatever belongs to your earthly nature . . . ." By the way, when we put something to death, it is best that we do not slowly torture it to death. "Put to death" or "rid yourself" is a swift, fast action. What we like to do, though, is think about it, consider giving up the food, hear other people talking about giving up their food, and check them out to be sure they have not died doing it—you know, the "drip-drip" method. We do not like to rush into things, but playing around with this process can only get us into real trouble. But as one thing dies, the life of God comes alive in our hearts!

The antagonist

Just as we see in literature a pattern of a hero or heroine opposed by an antagonist, we find in our own lives the existence of the True Hero and His antagonist. God's role is to give us truth, while Satan's role is to keep our minds confused and unfocused on God's ways. One way that Satan accomplishes this feat is through lies.

People who are especially vulnerable to these deceitful lies could be people who have not died to their own wills. When we do not die to our own will, we usually do not diagnose ourselves properly. We start blaming anything and everything around us as the sources of our unhappiness, or we become very depressed and even more deeply engrossed in self and filled with self-pity. This leads to more earthly comforts, such as overeating to soothe ourselves. People call this "just a cycle." I call it a "downward spiral," and we cannot even feel or see it.

Satan can lie to us, and if he stays around long enough, he can become our master without our even knowing it. He is very discreet. He does not want us to know that *he* is our lord. Look at this curious dialogue between Jesus and the preacher-teachers of the day in the Gospel of John. Jesus starts by telling them that neither God nor Abraham was their father. The Bible records their reply:

"We are not illegitimate children," they protested. "The only Father we have is God himself." Jesus said to them, "If God were your Father, you would love me, for I came from God and now am here. I have not come on my own; but he sent me. Why is my language not clear to you? Because you are unable to hear what I say. You belong to your father, the devil, and you want to carry out your father's desire. He was a murderer from the beginning, not holding to the truth, for there is no truth in him. When he lies, he speaks his native language, for he is a liar and the father of lies. Yet because I tell the truth, you do not believe me! Can any of you prove me guilty of sin? If I am telling the truth, why don't you believe me? He who belongs to God hears what God says. The reason you do not hear is that you do not belong to God." (John 8:41b–47)

The Pharisees (the preachers of Jesus' day) knew Scripture. They went to the temple constantly. However, their wills had not submitted to the will of the Heavenly Father. They were quickly adopted by the father of the dark world. If your will is to love God with all of your heart, your soul, and your mind, then you can hear His voice. But, if your will is to halfway serve Him when it is convenient, you will not hear His voice. You cannot hear His voice. Once again, you cannot have two masters.

We are all recovering Pharisees, or we have all known people who are like the Pharisees. Pharisees are uncomfortable in the presence of someone who has submitted his will. They avoid spiritual conversations, and the lifestyle and behavior of spiritual people often seem stupid to them. Pharisees might be the type who, when they go to worship, criticize the sermon, the song leaders, the people in the choir, the elders, the ministries, and the number of contributions. They have forgotten that the whole idea behind the Sunday morning gathering is *self-examination*. As I spend more

If your will is to love God with all of your heart, your soul, and your mind, then you can hear His voice.

and more time examining myself, I feel better and happier. My job description is not to help God fix other people, but to work on myself with the help of God.

All of us have our times when we resist having things go God's way. Even the beloved Apostle Peter, in Matthew 16:22–23, voiced the ways of Satan and not God when he said:

"Never, Lord!" he said. "This shall never happen to you!" Jesus turned and said to Peter, "Get behind me, Satan! You are a stumbling block to me; you do not have in mind the things of God, but the things of men."

At all times, we must keep the right mental attitude to win victory in the battles we face. If we have a heart for it, it will be easy.

Satan is the ruler of this world, we are told. That is why he was able to offer to Jesus the kingdoms of the world and their splendor, if Jesus would, as Satan put it, "bow down and worship me." Notice the way Jesus fought the spiritual battle and won victory over temptation and the way He eventually got rid of the tempter for a time.

He did it by quoting God's truths or telling the truth. You can read this in the fourth chapter of Matthew.

The strategy

Be alert

So we have been called to be soldiers in a battlefield. Your assignment, should you decide to accept it, is to fight your desire for food by being alert. Keep in mind that the very time of day when we finally let down and relax and want to reward ourselves with food for making it through such a hard day is the very time that we are to be in the watchtower, alert to the enemy. The times that we celebrate with food because something wonderful has happened are the times we actually must be very watchful, sober, and on our guard. The times when we seem bored, with nothing to do, when eating crosses our minds as a way to fill the day, are the very times that we must be most active and busy carrying out God's will and not our own. The time when we finally think everyone has gone to bed and no one is looking is the very time the room might be full of demons ready to lie to and torment us; but it is also filled with a great crowd of heavenly beings cheering us on to victory. And we are not even aware of it! I have spent most of my life asleep to the spiritual realm. "Wake up, O sleeper!" (Ephesians 5:14).

We know that we are children of God, and that the whole world is under the control of the evil one. (1 John 5:19)

Be self-controlled and alert. Your enemy the devil prowls around like a roaring lion looking for someone to devour. Resist him, standing firm in the faith, because you know that your brothers throughout the world are undergoing the same kind of sufferings.

And the God of all grace, who called you to his eternal glory in Christ, after you have suffered a little while, will himself restore you and make you strong, firm and steadfast. To him be the power for ever and ever. Amen. (1 Peter 5:8–11)

We are warned many times to be alert. I am convinced that every one of us is here to learn to raise our consciousness level to be alert to God every hour of the day. That is why your battles will be something different every day and at different hours. You are not going to have the same exams. Yet, Satan is good at making us believe that we are OK and that there are no battles. Or, on the other end of the spectrum, the "accuser of the brethren" makes us feel as though God does not love us. Not true! His tactics are to remain in the background and chip away at us, or have us lose the battles so subtly that we do not even know that we are in a battle— much less losing it—like a boat slowly drifting to the sea. His major goal is to distance you from God and from truth.

The times when we seem bored, with nothing to do, when eating crosses our minds as a way to fill the day, are the very times that we must be most active and busy carrying out God's will and not our own.

Beware of the Tempter's tactics

Look at what Satan has done with the weight loss world. He has encouraged dieting, and our flesh loved it because we did not have to take our heart off food, repent, change, or obey God. We have just made the food repent and change, and we have forced the whole food industry to change and manipulate our food. We have forced the restaurants to change what they are serving us. And very few people know it. Isn't that interesting! We have wrongly believed that external changes help us. Very few, even if they know better, have the nerve to stand up against this foolishness because the Pharisees of the weight loss world are so strong-headed and self-righteous about their broccoli, carrots, and low-fat foods when they are eating in public. After all, it is easier to clean up the outside than the inside.

Satan has made sure, in the meantime, that we believe we do not need to examine ourselves. Now, *there* is the problem. This pharisaical attitude (cleaning up the outside while the inside harbors dead men's bones) has even permeated our trusted research. Why, major industries and government agencies spend tons of money to research changing the food content for good health measures. They spend money for researching your genes and your brown and your white fat cells. They have suggested that all overweight is genetic and your mother's fault. This is really scary, because we have all believed this general labeling at one time or another. Yet, in all my years of starting people on Weigh Down*, I have observed that whenever someone ate less food, they lost weight—so they are not genetically condemned.

You really have to be on your toes to see the hand of Satan. He does not show up at your house in a red suit with a pitchfork. Satan and his insidious crew are such clever underground agents that they make it difficult for many of us, when we begin the Weigh Down Workshop*, to believe that we even are overeating—until our eyes are opened to see how little food it takes to live. The main tool he can use on us is the lie. But look what damage it has done over the centuries, starting with Eve in the Garden. " 'You will not surely die,' the serpent said to the woman. 'For God knows that when you eat of it your eyes will be opened, and you will be like God, knowing good and evil' " (Genesis 3:4,5). Or to paraphrase Satan—there is more . . . God is holding out on you—there is more!

Stand firm

Now you have most of the painted picture. We are at war. The battleground is located in the mind and heart. Our assignment is to put to death the deeds of the flesh and put in their place the precious, wonderful will of our Heavenly Father. Last, but not least, Satan has a vested interest in sabotaging the whole mission by using very clever, deceitful lies.

Now that you know the fundamentals, how can you survive and be victorious in warfare? It is going to take your strength—*spiritual strength*. Let us look at Ephesians 6:13–18:

> Therefore put on the full armor of God, so that when the day of evil comes, you may be able to stand your ground, and after you have done everything, to *stand*. *Stand firm* then, with the

belt of truth buckled around your waist, with the breastplate of righteousness in place, and with your feet fitted with the readiness that comes from the gospel of peace. In addition to all this, take up the shield of faith, with which you can extinguish all the flaming arrows of the evil one. Take the helmet of salvation and the sword of the Spirit, which is the word of God. And pray in the Spirit [which means praying for what God wants and not what your flesh wants] on all occasions with all kinds of prayers and requests. With this in mind, be alert and always keep on praying for all the saints.

Once again, Paul warns us to be alert. And you thought all you had to do today was to go into work, try to please the boss, then go home, cook supper, prop up your feet, and watch the news. That is exactly what the enemy wants us to think! No, you must have an alert heart and mind looking for what pleases God, and be ready for the attack. When you hear the lie, quote the truth and then stand firm and watch God fight the battle.

A typical battle

Let us walk through a typical daily battle. You have just come home for the day, you are physically tired, and three old lies pop into your head:

Lie #1: You have made it through a tough day at work; therefore, you deserve to eat food.

Lie #2: When you are physically tired, the food will make you feel better.

Lie #3: You have so much to lose, what does it matter? You may as well eat when you are not hungry.

There you have it. The battleground and the test are set up for you, specifically for you. You are standing in front of the refrigerator and you feel this overwhelming, magnetic pull toward the food. Here is what you should do.

1. *Identify the lies and quote the truth.* The first strategic move is to get out of the kitchen and immediately identify the lies of Satan. Note the time you begin this battle. Quote the truth against the lie. The truth is that eating is not something we *deserve* to

do; it is something we are to do when and because we are
hungry. Food makes us feel worse, not better, if we are not
hungry. And the amount of weight we have to lose is not the

It is really
hard even to
know what
God's will is
until we have
a broken and
contrite
heart . . . .

criterion which we use for whether we are going to be obedient. Tell Satan we are to obey
the Lord, our God. Matthew 4:4 says, "Man
does not live on bread alone, but on every word
that comes from the mouth of God."
Many times Satan does not even have to hang
around. After all, he talked us into believing
these lies some years ago when he started us
out on our first so-called "deserved overindulgence." Since everyone else in America seemed
to be doing it and endorsing it, then we did
not even put up a fight. After many years of
overindulging, it has become what we call a
"stronghold," and this is very serious business.

2. *Get on your knees and submit your will to God.* Tell Him what
your desire is, and be honest. Say, "God, what I want to do is
to go to the refrigerator and eat the rest of the leftover turkey—
and the dressing—and some ice cream—to be exact, approximately a half-gallon! And I am pretty sure that if I get started,
I will probably finish off the rest of the homemade chocolate
pie. At least that is what I want to do. But I know that Your
will is for me not to eat a bite of this until my body calls for it.
I submit my head hunger or desires to Your will, not mine. I
am learning that what You are having me do is life, life, *life,*
and peace. And God, I realize I have been following Satan's
lies and my will, and that is miserable. It has gotten me nowhere but in trouble. So, please, take this desire away and give
me a 'full' feeling from You."

3. *Submit, and eat less food.* Use your remaining strength to determine that when you walk out of your bedroom, you are not
going to eat until you feel a growl. You will then start to feel
your prayer being answered or the magnetic force of food ending, to the point that you do not even want to eat. You cannot
even imagine wanting to eat the food. God has heard your

prayer and has taken the desire away and your heart starts feeling happy. One hour later, you fit into an outfit that you have not been able to get into for years!

Again, note the time on your watch. You can expect your battles to become less time-consuming as you become more practiced in submitting your will. I know that my battles can last anywhere from ten minutes to an hour, depending on how quickly I go through the steps.

Write these three steps down on your bathroom mirror or on your refrigerator. Memorize them for life. The problem with our battles is that we feel so confused and emotional while we are fighting them. But if you follow these steps, watch how the layers of confusion clear up.

It is really hard even to know what God's will is until we have a broken and contrite heart—a deeply sorrowful heart, as shown in Isaiah 66:2b, "'This is the one I esteem: he who is humble and contrite in spirit, and trembles at my word.' "

By the way, *contrite* means "sorrowful to the point of repentance or change." The main thing to know is: the quicker you give up your will, the sooner the battle will be over. Once you have truly determined never to give in to food again, the less Satan will even tempt you in that area. Eventually, you will be out of the battle zone for food—and what a glorious day it is to announce perfect peace with food!

Review

Let us review. First, identify the lie and then remind yourself of the truth. Satan knows he has won if you do not know why you are in battle or what your defense is. Once you have determined this, you are not so emotional and out of control, but you are still confused. You wonder about how to handle this desire for food, because your will remains in the way. You wonder where full is and whether this is *head* or *stomach* hunger. Your will in the way clogs the arteries to life. You are dying, and you do not even know it. Satan has deceived us all into worrying about our cholesterol levels and plaque formations so much that no one even knows that it is our stubborn, adhesive, clogging will that causes the slow "death" from the lack of God's perfect, life-giving, free-flowing will into our life.

That is the second step—getting your will out of the way and just giving in to God's will. The less you have done this in life, the harder this will be. But remember—it is a choice. This step may bring tears to your eyes as you look to God and ask why He made life so hard. I have decided that is how our will is spilled out—through our tear ducts. One night I called a friend in the Weigh Down Workshop† to ask her how she was doing. I must have caught her in the middle of a struggle with her will, because she told me, "I'm just sitting here on the floor in front of my refrigerator and crying!" I asked if she had gotten anything from it to eat, and when she said no, I told her that she was doing fantastic; she did not have to be crying, for she was pleasing God. She had confronted her own will and was going through the painful process of putting it to death.

The third step, again, is to determine that you will not eat until your stomach growls.

The spoils of victory

The really neat thing about giving up the will is that it gets easier and easier if you repeat the process consistently, over and over. Once a big blockage of your will breaks loose, you experience life like you have never felt it. You will want to submit more and more as peace and happiness rush all through your veins. Quality sleep is abundant, and peace with food is more common than not. But best of all are the rewards, or the jewels, that you will get from your newfound ability to see and carry out His will.

God will always reward you for being obedient. Many incredible gifts will come from your victory. Many, many jewels have been reported for obedience. These are things that only God and you know you want very much. As you obey, He will give them to you. For example, we know many women who have reported finally becoming pregnant, parents whose children gave their lives to God, and people who did not have resources to buy new wardrobes, but who received clothes that would fit them each time they went down dress or pants sizes. You cannot explain away all the thousands of jewels such as these reported to our office.

You will never pursue another path once you have found the right one. Being skinny will only be a side benefit, certainly not the major reward for being obedient in this area of food. Once you go through this battle of the will, an incredible thing happens to all the confusion. It is like the scales that fell from Paul's eyes on the road to Damascus (see Acts 9). The confusion disappears, and you see clearly your way to God's will. It will be clear when to start eating and when to quit.

Another magnificent thing happens as the will for food is replaced with a will for God: you not only see God's will, but now you experience what He intended for you from the beginning of time. You *want* to do God's will. Do you see what I am saying? See, I *want* to eat in the same way I have been describing to you. I have been eating this way for fourteen years. Thin eating is fun. You could not pay me to overeat, because God has replaced my heart for food with a heart for Him. Every time you find the mystery of God's will and submit your own—fully, that is—it will be clear to you what to do. Eventually, God will transform your mind and heart so that you enjoy doing it His way. Having one mind brings much peace.

Conclusion

I have seen many people struggle when they realize that they have to give up their will. Many times, I have cried out to God that His system is too hard. God puts us through a tough course to surrender to His Spirit of love. He is a demanding professor and gives no easy pop quizzes in His classroom. Paul spoke of the training process in these terms:

> Not that I have already obtained all this, or have already been made perfect, but I *press* on to take hold of that for which Christ Jesus took hold of me. Brothers, I do not consider myself yet to have taken hold of it. But one thing I do: Forgetting what is behind and *straining* toward what is ahead, I *press* on toward the goal to win the prize for which God has called me heavenward in Christ Jesus. (Philippians 3:12–14)

And again, in 1 Corinthians 9:24–27, Paul wrote:

Do you not know that in a race all the runners run, but only one gets the prize? *Run in such a way as to get the prize.* Everyone who competes in the games goes into strict training. They do it to get a crown that will not last; but we do it to get a crown that will last forever. Therefore I do not run like a man running aimlessly; I do not fight like a man beating the air. No, *I beat my body* and make it my slave so that after I have preached to others, I myself will not be disqualified for the prize. I have always told people in the Weigh Down[†] seminars that your will rises up in the middle of the night like yeast-dough bread, and you must punch it or beat it back down by getting on your knees every morning.

So, again—passing God's pop quizzes is hard. But once you get through a few quizzes, knowing how to pass them will become much easier and much clearer. If you approach the battle fully prepared, using all your heart, soul, mind, and strength, the victory will be easier than when you are half-cocked or unprepared.

Remember, when you feel this ungovernable compulsion to over-eat, wake up and turn to God. As you battle, remember that there are heavenly hosts cheering you on, and that the victory over Satan and the worldly desires has been won. Do not even get out of bed now without putting on your full battle armor. Run so as to get the prize, which includes loving God with all of your strength! I have given God my strength, and He renews me daily. I am infinitely better off for surrendering my strength for His service and being energized for life's tasks with His strength.

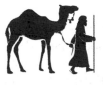

FEASTING ON THE WILL OF THE FATHER

Love the Lord with all of your soul . . .

Y ou may be halfway across the desert by now. For most of us this journey is not easy, but it is worthwhile. It is a bittersweet experience. In fact, there have been many hard days. In this place of sacrifice, we feel like we have given our mind, heart, and strength to God and yet something still seems to be wrong. Our weight seems to be stuck so that we are no longer losing. What is wrong?

Is it possible that God is asking for the last ingredient—our very soul—the eternal part of our being?

The easy times

My relationship with God was, in the beginning, like a newborn baby's with his mother. The mother feeds the baby, keeps the baby warm, keeps the baby clean, changes the baby's diaper, and keeps the baby distracted and happy. The baby does not have to do anything. The mother is "everything" to the baby.

But as time goes on, the baby grows and there is a response expected from the baby: obedience . . . attentiveness . . . love.

In the beginning, God was this "everything" for me and I just received. As I got older, God expected something back. It is not hard to give Him small things. However, by the time I had reached my late twenties and early thirties, I felt like I was in the heat of the desert. I could hardly believe how difficult the tests from God were and how much He was asking for then. To give to those who did not give back and to love those who did not love me back ran counter to the very core of my being and were going to require my very soul to accomplish. It seemed like pressure and difficulties came from all directions.

To get me to do His will, I felt as if God was going to have to "kill" the Gwen in me. With tears, I would ask God if He wanted a zombie for a follower. I asked Him if He wanted robots. I would reason with Him and remind Him that He already had angels who were made to do His will. Why did He make humans with a will, but ask them to die to their wills? I always ask questions with respect and with the intent to do things His way. At the time, I got no answers. Just trust and obey was what I had to cling to.

The last ten pounds

The Weigh Down† approach teaches us that we have to face little deaths to ourselves daily. For example, if we have desire eating and we want to eat before we go to bed, we must run to the opposite end of the house (away from the food), get down on our knees, die to our wishes, and ask God to remove this desire. This form of obedience involves *death to self*. Death to self, or our will, is the core of obedience.

obedience

Concern for self was the major emphasis of the Israelites.

"If only we had died by the Lord's hand in Egypt! There we sat around pots of meat and ate all the food we wanted, but you have brought us out into the desert to starve this entire assembly to death." (Exodus 16:3)

Do you feel as if God has brought you out into this desert to starve you to death? Do you feel that the amount of food He allows daily is way too small? Do you feel that the length of time between hunger signals is way too long? Do you feel that your spouse's love toward you is too little? Do you feel the financial situation God has left you in is too hand-to-mouth? Do you feel that the job God has handed you is not fulfilling enough? Do you despise this seemingly too skimpy lifestyle and have-to dependence on God's hand to control when you eat, how much money you have coming in, and how kind your spouse will be to you? Do you find this Desert of Testing to be unenjoyable while others applying Weigh Down Workshop[†] principles seem to be having a swell time? Have you been tempted, as the Israelites were, to go back to Egypt (the world), reasoning that at least on diets you could lust over food and chew on optional calories when you wanted to chew? At least in Egypt, you did not have a tug of war with your heart. You could let your heart just love the food by bingeing out. The thought of letting loose and saving yourself from "death" is tempting.

You have lost twenty pounds, but now the amount of food you have cut back to only leaves you at a plateau. You know you have ten more pounds to go. God seems to want more from you. In fact, He wants some of the last morsels that you thought were rightfully yours. Have you not given enough? It is like people working on marriage relationships. Some of you feel you have given up so many of your rights to make your partner happy and marriage is better, but God seems to ask you to die to your wishes even more! How could this be when you feel like justice would require your spouse, for once, to die to his or her wishes for the sake of peace! God is asking the person who seems to be the doormat to exhibit even more willingness to be trampled. God is asking the person who gives his coat to give his jacket, too. God is asking us to turn the other cheek after one has been slapped.

From Paradise to suffering

If you are like me, you would at least like to know why we have to suffer to the point of death to our own wills. Why is God asking for

our very soul to be sacrificed on the altar or for us to follow the steps
of Jesus all the way to the cross with this food? Can we not hold on
to some of our will?

> To this you were called, because Christ suffered for you, leaving
> you an example, that you should follow in his steps. "He com-
> mitted no sin, and no deceit was found in his mouth." When
> they hurled insults at him, he did not retaliate; when he suf-
> fered, he made no threats. Instead, he entrusted himself to him
> who judges justly. He himself bore our sins in his body on the
> tree, *so that we might die* to sins and live for righteousness . . . . (1
> Peter 2: 21–24)

He died so that we might die. Most of us are taught that when we
come to Christ, He has done all the dying. The walk with God tells
us differently.

When God started off with Adam and Eve, His obvious intent
was to provide mankind with a life free of worry, sacrifice, suffering, and death. But what quickly became apparent through Adam
and Eve's behavior was that man's heart did not consider Paradise
"good enough."

They mistakenly thought there had to be greener grass "out there"
somewhere. They made one major mistake. They did not recognize
true happiness when they saw it, so they figuratively traded the
brand new car for what was behind door number three. When they
saw what was behind door number three, a fallen world, I am sure
that they had a really sick feeling in their stomachs and could have
kicked themselves for failing to realize that there is nothing greater
than being with God.

God is now going to take us to the desert (the opposite of Paradise) with Him to test our heart and develop our heart of love for
Him. Our eyes will be opened to how great it is to be in favor with
God—even though we are in the heat of the desert. The environment will not matter once He is in your heart. After that, He will
hand us a "paradise" in the form of the Promised Land.

It seems that this new appreciation and character that Adam and
Eve needed was going to include pain, unfortunately; for God saw
that unless His children experienced pain, they did not seem to ap-
preciate freedom from pain. Without the night we would not recog-

nize the day. Too much sunshine without rain makes a desert. After the fall, life was going to be tougher.

Growing pains

Job said, "Shall we accept good from God, and not trouble?" (Job 2:10). It is a given that we will suffer. It is a given that God will discipline us if we need it. 1 Peter 4:12,13 says,

Dear friends, do not be surprised at the painful trial you are suffering, as though something strange were happening to you. But rejoice that you participate in the sufferings of Christ, so that you may be overjoyed when his glory is revealed.

This advice is certainly not what we hear from our mothers, friends, counselors, psychologists, psychiatrists, or our hair dressers! Think of a situation at work or in your marriage that casts you in the role of the underdog. Did your friends and colleagues make you focus only on yourself as the victim? Did they make you feel like it was something strange happening to you, and that you needed to take care of yourself? The world will tell you emphatically that you must indulge or take care of yourself, for no one else will. That lie has permeated even the church and is one of the biggest lies of Satan. But the Apostle Peter says not to be surprised when you suffer, and it is not *if* you will suffer but *when* you will suffer.

Nothing is strange about suffering being a part of the lot of our life, and nothing is strange about not wanting to suffer. But Jesus said that there was a cost to embracing his lifestyle. "And anyone who does not carry his cross and follow me cannot be my disciple" (Luke 14:27). There are some people who do not even know they are to pick up their cross, and there are some people who put their crosses down or even put their crosses on the backs of others. But this verse says that they cannot be a Christ-follower, a Christian, a disciple of Jesus, if they are not willing to pick up suffering or self-denial (the same thing) and carry it with them. Christ's followers must be willing to embrace pain—there is no backing out. And the pain *is* painful! Hebrews 12:11a tells us, "No discipline seems pleasant at the time, but painful." Suffering is not unique to you; it is normal, but it is painful.

Your cross, by the way, is not your mother-in-law. She is an opportunity for you to show love, not a cross to bear. Bearing your cross means laying down your will and doing God's. Even Jesus prayed with sweat drops of blood as He surrendered His will to God's: "Not my will but yours be done" (Luke 22:42).

God made us one way by nature. "Surely I was sinful at birth, sinful from the time my mother conceived me" (Psalm 51:5). Yet He asks, calls, or destines us to go another way. To embrace changing our self is to embrace growing pains. Just like children, we too were programmed to desire to grow up, but the intermittent pain that comes with accepting more responsibility is uncomfortable. However, staying immature is even more painful.

How to face giving up the food

Know that it is God's oven

Everything that happens to you from Satan is screened by God first. This dialogue between Satan and God assures us that God is in control. When you are threshed like wheat (tested), it is only by God's permission. Look at this passage from Job 1:7–12.

The LORD said to Satan, "Where have you come from?" Satan answered the LORD, "From roaming through the earth and going back and forth in it."

Then the LORD said to Satan, "Have you considered my servant Job? There is no one on earth like him; he is blameless and upright, a man who fears God and shuns evil."

"Does Job fear God for nothing?" Satan replied. "Have you not put a hedge around him and his household and everything he has? You have blessed the work of his hands, so that his flocks and herds are spread throughout the land. But stretch out your hand and strike everything he has, and he will surely curse you to your face."

The LORD said to Satan, "Very well, then, everything he has is in your hands, but on the man himself do not lay a finger." Then Satan went out from the presence of the LORD.

At the end of this testing, Job learned that the all-powerful God of the Universe holds the answer to suffering. Job argued to God that he was sinless and not deserving of suffering. God finally spoke and put Job in his place by asking him a few questions that he could not answer, such as "Where were you when I laid the earth's foundation?" (Job 38:4). Job understood then that we may not have all the answers to why we suffer. "Surely I spoke of things I did not understand, things too wonderful for me to know" (Job 42:3).

There is one major lesson to know or you will not be able to face the death to self: it is the necessity of experiencing God's cooking pot. If you are cooking out in this desert, it is under the auspices of the Heavenly Father. He knows how to get each pot to the correct temperature so as to melt off impurities from our hearts. If you believe you are a victim, that God is picking on you, or that you should not suffer because it is time for someone else to suffer, then you might jump out of the cooking pot, out of the hot desert, or off the altar. Ezekiel 24:3b–5 says:

The only thing that can possibly make me stay in this heat is to know that it is God's oven.

> " 'Put on the cooking pot; put it on and pour water into it. Put into it the pieces of meat, all the choice pieces —the leg and the shoulder. Fill it with the best of these bones; take the pick of the flock. Pile wood beneath it for the bones; bring it to a boil and cook the bones in it.' "

The only way I have ever been able to tough it out is to know that this pressure to submit my will is from the Father. James 1:2–4 points out, "Consider it pure joy, my brothers, whenever you face trials of many kinds, because you know that the testing of your faith develops perseverance. Perseverance must finish its work so that you may be mature and complete, not lacking anything." Most of us have been through some significant suffering. Some have suffered child abuse, sexual abuse, or molestation. Others have experienced verbal abuse, injustice, and financial devastation. We have all endured many things, no matter what it looks like on the outside.

It sounds all well and good that we will gain so much patience

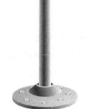

YOUR WAY
Get revenge, reward, or save yourself first.

Pain, an unsettled heart, and consequences come later.

GOD'S WAY
Endure pain first.

Rewards and peace come later from God.

and character, but when I am in the middle of having to give up my food or my way, gaining more character is no motivation for me. As I said before, the only thing that can possibly make me stay in this heat is to know that it is God's oven. Because He is so coordinated, so worthy of respect, such a great CEO of the Universe, I would not consider running from the desert if that is where He wants me. I would consider changing only my will and desires.

For example, even if a marriage is tough—God hates for you to jump out of the cooking pot before the cooking is done. God and Jesus always encouraged us first to stay in the oven!

Change yourself before you change the surroundings. Make sure God is leading you to change jobs, or God just might re-create the same situation in the next job. Do not even think about getting even with someone who has wronged you—in fact, turn the other cheek.

How do I know if I am right about this? Just try it for yourself. Try to get out of any suffering, including the painful suffering of dying to yourself with food. You will find that you remain miserable. And if you jump out of one cooking pot or off the altar, you will find that God will put you in another. You seemingly will put on five pounds overnight, and you will feel downcast again. Now reverse that choice of behavior and just bear through the wait for hunger. You will come through the pain and feel fantastic on the other side. You will get on the scales and reap reward! It boils down to the illustration above.

Jesus suffered

Another way that I have been able to endure the pain of change is to know that even Jesus did not escape the suffering, and He was God's favorite, so to speak. Hebrews 5:7–10 refers to the suffering that Jesus bore. "During the days of Jesus' life on earth, he offered up prayers and petitions with loud cries and tears to the one who could save him from death, and he was heard because of his reverent submission. Although he was a son, he learned obedience from what he suffered and, once made perfect, he became the source of eternal salvation for all who obey him and was designated by God to be high priest . . . ." So, even Jesus suffered. Isaiah expressed it very well:

> Yet it was the LORD's will to crush him and *cause him to suffer* and though the LORD makes his life a guilt offering, he will see his offspring and prolong his days, and the will of the LORD will prosper in his hand. After the suffering of his soul, he will see the light of life and be satisfied. (Isaiah 53:10,11a)

The words of Isaiah came true. After the suffering, He saw the light of life and was satisfied. Obviously, acknowledging Jesus' willingness to suffer helps us swallow this bitter pill.

So, not only do we endure the sufferings sent by God—we offer ourselves to suffering as God calls for it because it says to the world, "I believe and trust that this is a good God with great ability to run the world." When we endure and allow this outward suffering, others will witness the inside of us being very much alive, beautiful, and valuable. Happiness is something made on the inside of you.

Jesus suffered and voluntarily gave His life because the Father asked this of Him.

The products of suffering

> Therefore, I urge you, brothers, in view of God's mercy, to offer your bodies as living sacrifices, holy and pleasing to God—this is your spiritual act of worship. (Romans 12:1)

God has placed so much symbolism for death on this physical earth. Let me try to explain this paradox by some illustrations.

A caterpillar essentially "dies" in its cocoon so
that a butterfly can emerge. Consider the spring
that follows a harsh, deadly winter. Every
year we watch trees lose their leaves, appearing to die; yet they come back to life
bigger and stronger than before. Another symbol of life from death
around us is the daily example of
the long, cold night and the warmth
of the morning sun rising again. We
have to believe that the sun will rise
again. Jesus drew a great word picture for us:

> "I tell you the truth, unless a kernel of wheat falls to the ground
> and dies, it remains only a single seed. But if it dies, it produces
> many seeds. The man who loves his life will lose it, while the
> man who hates his life in this world will keep it for eternal life.
> Whoever serves me must follow me; and where I am, my ser-
> vant also will be. My Father will honor the one who serves me."
> (John 12:24–26)

God wants to build our faith in the idea that life comes from death.
If we stay in the cooker, it will dissolve the self-will. If we live and
die in the little ways and watch Him give us jewels, character or
rewards of any kind after obedience, then we will be able to handle
physical death with faith that He is going to take care of us. Then we
can truly say with the prophet Hosea, "Where, O death, are your
plagues? Where, O grave, is your destruction?" (Hosea 13:14b). It
was rephrased by Paul in 1 Corinthians 15:55, " 'Where, O death, is
your victory? Where, O death, is your sting?' "

God does not want us to be empty bodies without personalities
or original ideas. When we die to our will and get off the throne—
He puts His great personality (Holy Spirit) in its place. We become
unified and married, so to speak. "The two shall become one." What
a fantastic mystery!

He does not want a zombie, but rather a willing servant. This is
delicate surgery, and God will not let it go so deep that it kills the
very spirit that He is trying to transform. God is performing this
delicate surgery of stretching your heart into immortal character. It

is somewhat like the artistry of blown glass. If the glass is blown and stretched too hard or too fast, it may break apart. God does not want to stretch our hearts to the point that we break apart; rather, He wants our hearts to grow. The rain showers in our life, when we have to stretch to navigate the puddles, prepare us for the big storms.

We do not need to blame God or get angry at the training of God. After all, God created this "Life from Death University," and He created the students. Jesus is the Great Professor because He lived out the instructions we should live by.

I would say that the unity that comes from submerging our will into His will is the biggest allure to the suffering and death to self, in that it helps transform us to no longer desire overeating or any other worldly desire. There is no more internal strife or battles—just peace, deep peace.

We do have natural tendencies, or temptations, to jump out of this Desert of Testing. When the cooking pot gets to boiling temperatures, we often quit. I know. I have been in the boiler many times because my own will is so stubborn. We can resist the hand of God and wind up no better for all the pain that we have been through. Such was the plight of the Israelites referred to in Ezekiel 24:10–13:

> So heap on the wood and kindle the fire. Cook the meat well, mixing in the spices; and let the bones be charred. Then set the empty pot on the coals till it becomes hot and its copper glows so its impurities may be melted and its deposit burned away. It has frustrated all efforts; its heavy deposit has not been removed, not even by fire.
>
> " 'Now your impurity is lewdness. Because I tried to cleanse you but you would not be cleansed from your impurity, you will not be clean again until my wrath against you has subsided.' "

This is not a pretty picture. Oh, our stubborn hearts! God wants so badly for us to understand His ways and His love for us, but we have some wild, untamed hearts. We are bucking stallions that need to submit to the rider's hand. Once we understand God's rules, we can be guided left and right and be allowed to gallop full speed ahead. We are like some of the trees in the fall that refuse to drop their leaves, until a strong November blast removes them. We must yield to His hand. Then we develop the faith to die more and more. None of us has suffered for God so much that we have lost blood. "In your struggle against sin, you have not yet resisted to the point of shedding your blood" (Hebrews 12:4). At almost every public presentation when I address an audience, I ask them, "Do I look dead from dying to my will? No! I look alive!" Do the people in this book who have lost 100 pounds of their will look dead? No, alive! Life comes from death!

That dying produces life is a mystery that confounds the world, but it is the mystery that sets Christianity apart from other religions. And there is a difference between self-selected self-denial just for the praise of man and denial decided by God and accepted because you trust God. Following this path that Jesus walked will bring life to every fiber of your soul.

God wants your soul. All I want to tell you is that life comes from death in such a powerful way. The suffering that we go through to give Him our very soul does not compare to the glory that we enjoy.

When Jesus was in His darkest hour, on the cross with the nails in His hands and feet, feeling forsaken by God, witnesses to the crucifixion called out to Him *save yourself . . . save yourself . . . save yourself.* (See Luke 23.) *Save yourself* will be the overwhelming temptation when you are giving up more food, being falsely accused by a family member, church member, or co-worker. You will be tempted to take care of yourself and remove yourself from the altar. But if you give in to the temptation, you will miss the incredible work and rescue of the Mighty Warrior and Savior, our God. You will miss it!

God calls us to offer our bodies as living sacrifices, but we keep crawling off the altar, jumping out of the cooking pot, or rolling off the surgery table. Do we not know that we will live even more? The answer is to remember Jesus . . . "As the time approached for him to be taken up to heaven, Jesus resolutely set out for Jerusalem" (Luke 9:51).

Jesus resolutely set out to obey God and face the death He was called to. We must resolutely set out and face Jerusalem—death to this desire to eat. For Jesus said, "The reason my Father loves me is that I lay down my life—only to take it up again" (John 10:17). If you do not, you will miss feasting on the will of the Father.

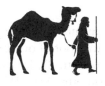

LOVE YOUR NEIGHBOR
AS YOURSELF

W e have learned in Phase II that, above all else, we must love God with all our heart, mind, soul, and strength. But the rest of this commandment from God that follows closely behind is *love your neighbor as yourself.*

We do love ourselves

We have had several decades of teachers and counselors feeding the population the untruth that people do not love themselves. Most people I have counseled in the Weigh Down Workshop[†] had been told their problems arose from not caring for themselves and taking time for themselves. The solution that had been suggested was: learn to love yourself, care for yourself, pamper yourself, and take time for yourself. Many advisors have suggested that this tends to affect women more than men because women are, by nature, care givers, and they find themselves doing a lot for others—as if this is a problem! People are taught to make sure they indulge themselves with TV, sports, beer, and fast cars. "Grab all the gusto you can get! After all, no one else is going to look out for you."

By now, I am sure it does not surprise you that "I protest!" The
world has misdiagnosed the root of our problems again.

First, I believe that we do naturally love ourselves. We feed, clothe,
wash, and spend money on ourselves. We hide food for and worry
about ourselves. In fact, we love ourselves very much; we can get
down because we obsessively think about ourselves, overfeed ourselves, and spend too much for our clothing. We buy all the latest
skin products, cosmetics and extra toiletries to pamper ourselves.
We spend too much money on ourselves, and we horde food to the
exclusion of our own children. We adore "Number One" too much!

Why do you think Jesus told us to love our neighbor as ourselves
if we were not programmed by God at birth to love ourselves? Look
at this passage from Ephesians where husbands are instructed to
love their wives:

> In this same way, husbands ought to love their wives as their
> own bodies. He who loves his wife loves himself. After all, *no
> one ever hated his own body,* but he feeds and cares for it, just as
> Christ does the church — for we are members of his body. (Eph-
> esians 5:28–30)

Second, it is a blessing—not a problem—to be a care giver by nature. People who truly do this for the Lord are renewed, not dis-
tressed; for when you focus on God and others, He takes care of
your needs. As we have said before, the flesh inside us loves the
"save yourself" cry from Satan and his demonic team, while Jesus
quietly whispers, "There is a God, a good God." In fact, the teachings that Jesus brought us from the Father cry out the opposite of
the world's teachings, so much so that you almost have to do a
double-take when you read the Bible.

> "Blessed are the poor in spirit, for theirs is the kingdom of heaven.
> Blessed are those who mourn, for they will be comforted.
> Blessed are the meek, for they will inherit the earth.
> Blessed are those who hunger and thirst for righteousness, for
>   they will be filled . . . .
> Blessed are those who are persecuted because of righteousness,
>   for theirs is the kingdom of heaven." (Matthew 5:3-6,10)

"Do *not* save yourself," the Word of God cries out, like a voice in the
wilderness. What God calls us to is the opposite of world thinking.

Even churches that supposedly uphold the "old rugged cross" offer "How to Build Self-Esteem" and "How to Love Yourself More" seminars. Yet, the Bible teaches that self-love is a given, and that *self-denial* is also a part of the will of the Father. If we have made Him happy, then we will be at peace with ourselves. Obedience to God is the key to self-esteem, for it brings acceptance of God to our heart. If the God of the universe is for us, who could possibly be against us?

Love others—do not blame others

Since we do love ourselves, we need to take those actions of love that we give ourselves and give them to someone else, too. As Jesus said, "Love your neighbor as yourself." Show concern for them, feed them, clothe them, and care for them. Then we will like ourselves more. Do not take the bad advice to pamper yourself, because you will despise your overly self-indulgent actions.

After all, no one ever hated his own body, but he feeds and cares for it . . . (Ephesians 5:28)

Overly focusing on self provides only temporary delight and ultimately leaves a bad taste in the mouth. It also turns other people off, so that you become more isolated. We have tried it—it does not work!

The world cries out that you will not lose weight until you love yourself, or, vice versa, you will not love yourself until you lose weight! People of the world say what you feel about yourself dictates whether you will have a good day. They say if you make taking care of "Number One" your sole priority, then you will have a good "eating" day. But I say, getting your focus off of self and onto God and obedience to Him will cause you to have a good "eating" day. If you love and trust the Lord, you will feed yourself the appropriate amount, and you will not indulge in desire eating. One day, you will look down to find that you have lost more and more weight! You will then be more in love with God for saving you from preoccupation with overly focusing on yourself. In other words, there is a healthy, appropriate focus on care of self. We tend to think if a little bit is good, then a lot is better; but, in the case of excessive self-love, it is empty and usually empties our pocketbooks. The balanced way leads to life; the other leads to death.

Usually, someone else is going to have to be blamed for our bad day. I am sorry to say that spouses and friends get the brunt of it. Usually, loved ones are the scapegoats. They are blamed for sabotaging you by offering regular food or inviting you to a birthday party!

Others are not to blame for sabotaging your eating. No one but you can make your heart love food. No fat farm with its sterile, temptation-free environment will make your heart desire less food. It is so sad that we have made our families suffer by our unloving actions and also by making them clean up the environment for us by keeping no tempting foods in the house. The cabinets are full at my house, and we work on keeping our hearts cleaned up. Therefore, it is rare that we take advantage of our freedom. Think about this. There are people working daily in the Godiva chocolate factories who never gain weight over the years. You could not pay them to overeat. Why? It is the heart and what you love. It is not the people around you or your surroundings that make you have a good or bad day. It is simply what is in your heart and what you have given your heart to.

Love God first

When you read the Ten Commandments (Exodus 20), you will see that the first four commandments are talking about a relationship between you and God, and the last six concern your relationships with people. It is obvious that the first three are relational, and, if you look closely, you will see that the fourth is as well.

The third command, "You shall not misuse the name of the Lord, your God," is relational in that God is telling us not to misuse His name by calling Him "Lord" when we don't submit to Him as our Master. You are going to confuse the *world* if you are bowing down to the refrigerator one minute and calling God "Lord" the next. The fourth command, to keep the Sabbath day holy, is relational, too. God is saying, "Look, there are seven days in a week. Set apart one of those days for just you and Me—I want your total heart, soul, mind and strength that day. Can you not give Me just one day out of seven if I am truly the object of your affection?!"

How much trouble is it to refrain from running to another idol if you are so in love with God? These are easy commandments from this wonderful God. We should praise Him that salvation (being able to enter His presence) is not performance-based. We just need to love Him, and we can do this! If you truly love, it is not a performance or a drama—it is simply natural. If your love is golf, how hard is it to go play a game? Would you call a game of golf work? Of course not. How hard is it to binge on food? When food is the object of your affection, bingeing is a delight. Then, may our hearts change so that anything that has to do with God is delightful.

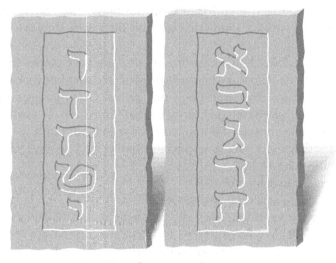

The Ten Commandments

1. You shall have no other gods before me.
2. You shall not make for yourself an idol... bow down to them or worship them....
3. You shall not misuse the name of the Lord your God....
4. Remember the Sabbath day by keeping it holy.
5. Honor your father and your mother...
6. You shall not murder.
7. You shall not commit adultery.
8. You shall not steal.
9. You shall not give false testimony against your neighbor.
10. You shall not covet....

Once you have the relationship in which God is your heart's desire, then, and only then, can you love mankind the way you should. That is why the commands to honor your father and mother, and not to murder, commit adultery, steal, give false testimony, or covet your neighbor's wife or anything of your neighbor's, are last—they are the natural outcomes of loving God first. If you love Him, how could you hurt one of the children that He loves? That would be unspeakable!

There are many people who love other people and have devoted their lives to mankind, but who do not love God. God said to love Him first—that is where your passion and strength and money should go. Loving your neighbor as yourself is different. You are not to worship your spouse, children, or other people. You worship only God, but this love for God will automatically spill over to loving the children God made. In fact, Scripture tells us that the way we know that we love God is by the love we show others.

Dear friends, let us love one another, for love comes from God. Everyone who loves has been born of God and knows God. Whoever does not love does not know God, because God is love . . . . Dear friends, since God so loved us, we also ought to love one another. No one has ever seen God; but if we love one another, God lives in us and his love is made complete in us. (1 John 4:7,8,11,12)

And again in John 15:9–17:

"As the Father has loved me, so have I loved you. Now remain in my love. If you obey my commands, you will remain in my love, just as I have obeyed my Father's commands and remain in his love . . . . My command is this: Love each other as I have loved you. Greater love has no one than this, that he lay down his life for his friends. You are my friends if you do what I command . . . . You did not choose me, but I chose you and appointed you to go and bear fruit —fruit that will last. Then the Father will give you whatever you ask in my name. This is my command: Love each other."

Sometimes our love for God naturally spills over to mankind, but sometimes we need to be commanded to love—even the unlovely.

Obviously, we will be closer to some people than others. Jesus had his favorite disciple; the Bible referred to the "disciple whom Jesus loved" (John 13:23).

Loving your neighbor includes loving your spouse. A bad relationship is a roadblock that can turn people to depression, anger, and rage, and send them running to food, wine, beer, and antidepressants.

Instead of trying to defend yourself . . .	*let God defend you.*
If you will give back kindness for unkindness . . .	*trust God to fill up the need you have.*
If you will repent of attempting to make others treat you right or do right . . .	*trust God to cover the poor decisions others make.*
If you will just love when you suffer unloving actions from others . . .	*expect God to love you back even more deeply.*

If we do all these things, we would straighten paths and build bridges so Christ could walk across to someone new. We and others around us would be so well taken care of if we would just try to surrender our rights first. Everything else will be added to us. Our children need to see this kind of faith in God. They will be taken care of, too. I have witnessed this truth. God defends us magnificently against our enemies like a dad who stands up for his child who is being treated unfairly. That is the heritage of those who love Him. Focus on God and obedience and off of self, and you will have better relationships.

> *If we do all these things, we would straighten paths and build bridges so Christ could walk across to someone new.*

The main problem with the theme of "I am doing what is best for me" is that it can strengthen the largest roadblock on the path to the Father—*pride*. The Bible clearly teaches us that God hates pride. Haughtiness is one of the seven deadly sins, according to the proverb:

There are six things the Lord hates, seven that are detestable to him: haughty eyes, a lying tongue, hands that shed innocent blood, a heart that devises wicked schemes, feet that are quick to rush into evil, a false witness who pours out lies and a man who stirs up dissension among brothers (Proverbs 6:16–19).

James gives you the answer to pride problems:

God opposes the proud but gives grace to the humble. Submit yourselves, then, to God. Resist the devil, and he will flee from you. Come near to God and he will come near to you. Wash your hands, you sinners, and purify your hearts, you double-minded. Grieve, mourn and wail. Change your laughter to mourning and your joy to gloom. Humble yourselves before the Lord, and he will lift you up (James 4:6b–10).

Humility is expecting nothing from mankind and looking to God to meet all your needs.

Once again, *you* humble yourself, and *He* will lift you up. You do not have to lift yourself. Humility is not being mousey or quiet. The Bible teaches us that "Moses was powerful in speech and action" (Acts 7:22), and God described him as "a very humble man, more humble than anyone else on the face of the earth" (Numbers 12:3). Humility is expecting nothing from mankind and looking to God to meet all your needs.

Do not try to get what you need from your spouse—expect nothing from man. Look to God for everything. In Him, you move and walk and have your being (Acts 17:28). Moses kept his eyes and heart on God—humility.

When you start loving God and it spills over to mankind, you will notice that it affects how you handle *your* food. For example, you might just cook some casseroles and send the biggest and best to your sick neighbor, whereas before, you kept the biggest and best for yourself. After potluck dinners, you used to take back your leftovers and would gladly take unclaimed leftovers, too. Now, you give all the leftovers away. In the past, you just could not bring yourself to part with your canned goods for the "canned food drives for the poor," but now you have faith that you can get more canned corn and tuna later.

Love God first and then your neighbor as yourself, and you will be taken care of. And who is your neighbor? Anyone God has placed in your way who has a need. And do not just halfway bandage them up—be like the good Samaritan and go all out with pouring out love and care and money on them.

These truths in this chapter make life worth living!

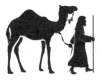

How to Measure Success

Many people start Weigh Down[†] and wonder how to measure whether they are successful. The scales may not be moving in the beginning, so they wonder if they are being "bad" or "good," or if they are being honest or dishonest with themselves.

Most other programs that you have been on are legalistic or full of rules. You know deep down that the rules are very hard to keep for any length of time. God has made it so that people cannot keep rules that their hearts do not accept.

As a result, you know deep down that you cannot stay on a diet. As you get older, you hate even to start another diet that you know you will not finish. The result of years of dieting is that you become accustomed to games and cheating and being dishonest with yourself. You go into the old diet programs, knowing exactly how to measure success. To the professional dieter, success is staying within the guidelines of a three-inch by three-inch piece of cornbread, half a cup of vegetables, a two-ounce piece of lean meat, and eight glasses of water. Perhaps cheating was when you ate a piece of birthday cake.

You also know exactly how you can cheat. You can fast before weigh-ins, eat all your free calories in one week, and use bigger serving spoons. And when you look at the food, your eyeball just gets bigger and bigger, so you say, "Yeah, I think that looks like a medium-sized potato" when it is really an extra-large potato. At weigh-ins (that dreaded time), you knew how to get that water weight off: starve yourself. I have known people who have gone so far as to remove their dentures before weigh-ins!

I can remember being on a food exchange diet program I learned while studying to be a dietitian. I remember being hungry at night after I had eaten all of my exchanges for the day. So I would just borrow food exchanges from the next day. By the end of the week, I had no food exchanges left. I had not gone by the rules. Besides, I was eating things that were not on the list. I considered myself successful when I stayed within the boundaries of the rules.

To the professional dieter, success is staying within the guidelines of a three-inch by three-inch piece of cornbread . . .

When you enter the Weigh Down Workshop[t], however, you are given such incredible freedom—with very few rules. Before, everything was already figured out for you. Now, you may feel pressure to make your own rules—and you may wonder if you are doing it right. It is easy to feel like a failure because of the lack of rules; if you are not hurting enough, you think you must be doing something wrong.

When you do not see the scales move, you panic. "Is this really hunger I'm feeling? Where is full? Can I eat one more bite? If I eat it, is this wrong? Am I just lying to myself or cheating again? I must be unsuccessful." So your heart cries out, "Teach me judgment! I am not used to this new system."

Let me start by saying that you may have been brainwashed all these years to think that success is a certain number of fat grams, or that cheating is when you have eaten a large piece of pizza. These rules are very burdensome and carry unnecessary guilt.

The Weigh Down Workshop[t] provides freedom in what you eat, but there is very clear structure that you are relearning. In the beginning, it may be very awkward, but your focus will grow stronger and stronger and become second nature as time goes by, unlike the burdensome rules of diets. In actuality, there is plenty of structure in the Weigh Down Workshop[†]. Yes, any food is OK, but just between the green light of hunger and red light of full. Just as sex outside of marriage creates havoc, and just as too many vacations and not enough work are unrewarding, so, too, food outside of hunger and fullness is not fulfilling. Sex is not wrong, vacations are not wrong, and birthday cake is not wrong, as long as they lie inside the context in which they were intended.

Sometimes "hunger" is unclear, but if you wait long enough, it becomes crystal clear. Sometimes "full" can be confusing. Even thin eaters make mistakes and go beyond full or eat when they do not feel true hunger. Do not be legalistic. When these thin eaters eat beyond full, they just wait for a strong hunger signal before they eat again, and they are right back on track. The object is to rid oneself of greed. If you do, the details will not matter.

Yes, even the thin eaters make mistakes, though I am sure these are the exceptions and not the rule; but they do not dwell on the mistakes. They just get right back on track. Likewise, you cannot start a heart change program and expect all the greed in your heart to rise to the surface overnight. Give it some time. God will be taking greed (feeding yourself) out a little at a time and replacing it with faith in His feeding ability. If you have lost ten pounds already, then it is possible that ten pounds of greed have already left your heart, never to return!

I do not want you toying with the idea of defeat, feeling unsuccessful, or giving up. I have seen so many people going through the Weigh Down Workshop[†] who are still trying to use their old guidelines to measure their success. About five weeks into the program, some of these people become depressed and feel guilty because they have not been keeping a Travel Diary (see Appendix D), and they feel like they have been "bad" all week long.

I tell these people that thin eaters do not necessarily keep a Travel Diary. There is no magic in any guidelines we have suggested. These guidelines are only provided in the hope that they might help you on this journey. They help you fall in love with God. Eventually you will only use your heart and stomach to guide you.

After explaining that important principle, I encourage them to let me decide whether they have been "bad" or not, since most of the participants have the wrong definition of "bad." I start to reprogram them by asking a few questions:

Q: Did you wait until you were hungry a few times this week?

A: Well, yes, but I did not use smaller plates.

Q: Never mind that. I am proud that you found hunger. Now, did you leave any food on your plate this week?

A: Well, yes. Come to think of it, I did that several times.

Q: Great! Well, all in all, did you eat a little less this week than you normally would have?

A: Well, yes, I did!

Q: Do you feel a little more in control as you focused on God instead of food?

A: Yes, yes, I think I see what you're getting at. Well, maybe I'm not so "bad" after all!

Of course this person is not bad! This person had a fantastic week. This person was not doing these things before the program. In fact, if most people think back to the time before they started the Weigh Down Workshop[†], they were starting a meal when they were full and stopping when they were painfully stuffed. In just a few short weeks, they have come to the point where they customarily eat smaller amounts of regular food. It brings back memories of their childhood eating when they enjoyed food. They may not have lost weight every week, but they have been successful in my eyes because they have started to change their behavior into that of a thin eater's.

This person is a success in God's eyes, and so are you. The heart, soul, mind, and strength are being given over to God in ways they never have before.

You probably could give me a whole list of wonderful heart changes, such as you found yourself thinking about food less often and you left one-fourth of a hamburger on your plate. Maybe you ate only half of a candy bar for the first time in your life. You found that you are not eating by the clock anymore. Before you started the program, you never allowed your body to empty out all the way to hunger, but now you do. You may have eaten beyond full this week, but you had never even perceived a stuffed stomach as being painful until this week. You ate some birthday cake, a nice-sized piece at that, but before the program you would not have stopped at a piece. You would not have stopped until you had cleared out two or three rows, or the entire cake.

You are a success because you have changed your heart's attitude toward food, and it is starting to affect the way you eat. You are a success because of behavioral changes. Even if you know there needs to be more trust in your heart that God is not going to starve you, your faith is increasing by your ability to give up a few more bites of this lunch or of that evening meal.

The victory is that you are now rating your food for the first time in your life. The changes are that you are conscious of your behavior and your amounts are smaller than before. The victory is that you sipped between bites. You looked up, it was 3:30, and you had not even thought about lunch. The plate of food you are now starting to eat looks enormous to you. Your stomach now seems to hold less food before it feels uncomfortable. You are leaving food behind when you feel satisfied; you are getting "picky" about every bite you put in your mouth, and you are using a regular glass instead of a sixty-four-ounce tumbler. And most of all, it now takes you fifteen minutes to eat fifteen M&Ms! You are just not pigging out as much as you used to. All in all, you are seeing definite heart, soul, mind, and strength changes.

At the same time, you feel more at peace. Someone at work said your face looks different, you are reading your Bible more, and you are communicating with God a lot more. Anger is leaving, and your marriage is better as you are able to love more and think about the needs of others more. You are starting to go through church doors again, and suddenly the preacher has improved his sermons. Even God's creation looks more beautiful—especially the sunsets.

Do you realize what is happening? You are making permanent heart changes, and each and every one of them is a change that leads to less food, less eating, more enjoyment of the food, and a permanent, thin you. These changes are something you can live with—

changes that become more natural every day. These changes shift the control of greed into your court. Food is starting to lose its control over you.

The only time you lose ground now is when you panic and look at the scales. In your weak moments, you think, "Oh, I have got to get this weight off faster," so you think you must go back on a diet. But I am asking you to take hold of yourself, get away from that temptation, and stay on the correct road of sure heart change. What you need to do is write down your positive behavior changes on your *Heart and Behavior Change List* (see the end of this chapter). Keep a copy of them posted on your bathroom mirror and use your scales less often. Show your behavior changes to your concerned relatives that are looking for (but not finding) low-fat foods in your refrigerator.

> *So success is when the heart changes, and then the body will follow.*

The ability to measure the heart's attitude toward food is not as visible or tangible as using scales or a measuring cup. Staying in the Word of God helps you have a standard to live by. God will make the heart feel bad if it is not in line. There are people this week that may have lost weight—but not because they have less greed in their heart. There are people who definitely are less greedy, but it did not show on the scales this week. Take inventory of your heart; the scales will eventually follow.

How quickly we forget! If you are one to forget quickly, put a bookmark in this chapter and read it daily. This attitude is an essential ingredient for success in this workshop. We must look deeper and relearn how to measure success in life. *What* you eat should not be your judge, but *how* you eat should. Small changes today will make tremendous changes six months or a year from now. Two years from now, the change will be even more dramatic. So, success is *not* measuring a three-inch by three-inch piece of cornbread. Success in the Weigh Down Workshop† is as simple as turning your heart toward God, and you can do this! It follows that your heart will turn away from the food. You will lose the weight as a side benefit. The major benefit will be knowing how good God is to us. The only mistake you can make in the Weigh Down Workshop[t] is to give up. Never give up, even if you are tempted to. I want everyone to reach this attainable goal. This is very important to me. All you have to do to be right back on track is to wait for the next hunger by calling out to God. It has helped many people in Weigh Down[t] to use a *Seek Ye First* list (see a sample at the end of this chapter).

We must seek God first in everything; we are told to "seek ye first the kingdom of God." Most of us have come so close as to "seek ye fifth" or "seek ye sixth." "Seek ye first" is not the instinct it should be. Once this habit is formed, though, it will make a great difference in the weight loss and your entire life. Keep preparing your heart.

So get away from the scales—a defeating and inaccurate tool to measure behavior change. Get away from self-defeating talk. Get away from unnecessary judgments that get you nowhere. Start today looking for heart and behavior changes that are occurring since you have started the Weigh Down Workshop[t] and make sure that you write all of these down on your list.

In summary, if measuring success is dependent upon the ability of the heart to change, then we should concentrate on the heart. This *attitude* will carry you to the completion of your weight-loss goals. So success is when the heart changes, and then the *body* will follow.

HEART AND BEHAVIOR CHANGE LIST

Write down your positive behavioral changes. Some changes will be emotional or mental, some will be spiritual, some will be related to your physical and spiritual strength, and some will be changes in weight. Think and write, and think and write. Let God open your eyes to how the Weigh Down[†] approach is affecting you and the people around you. You can use this, also, to list what God has done as you give your heart to Him.

Examples: *I'm desiring less food. I'm reading my Bible more.*

1. _____

2. _____

3. _____

4. _____

5. _____

6. _____

7. _____

8. _____

9. _____

10. _____

11. _____

12. _____

13. _____

14. _____

15. _____

Most of our desert storms are because we don't instinctively "seek God first." Instead of trying to do things or worry about things that are not a part of your job description from God—practice daily the following:

WEIGH DOWN WORKSHOP [†]

SEEK YE FIRST

Worries I give to God today

Areas of obedience to God

Things to do today

☐

☐

☐

☐

☐

☐

☐

☐

☐

☐

☐

☐

"Blessed is the man who listens to me, watching daily at my doors, waiting at my doorway. For whoever finds me finds life and receives favor from the LORD. But whoever fails to find me harms himself; all who hate me love death."

—Proverbs 8.34-36

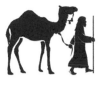

TRUE REPENTANCE

The Narrow Path

There are many outward manifestations of a heart not grounded on the Rock. Lists abound in the New Testament which show that the acts of the sinful nature start in our very own heart and mind. "Furthermore, since they did not think it worthwhile to retain the knowledge of God, he gave them over to a depraved mind, to do what ought not to be done. They have become filled with every kind of wickedness, evil, greed and depravity. They are full of envy, murder, strife, deceit and malice. They are gossips, slanderers, God-haters, insolent, arrogant and boastful; they invent ways of doing evil; they disobey their parents; they are senseless, faithless, heartless, ruthless" (Romans 1:28–31).

These compulsive behaviors can manifest themselves in unloving attitudes toward others or manifest themselves in outward displays of the flesh. To be true, one manifestation seems to be more visible. For example, the Prodigal Son types outwardly show greed, sensual indulgence, laziness, etc. It is there for the world to see. Then there are the older brother types who look like they are doing everything right on the outside—on time, productive, disciplined—but on the inside the personality characteristics are hateful, unloving,

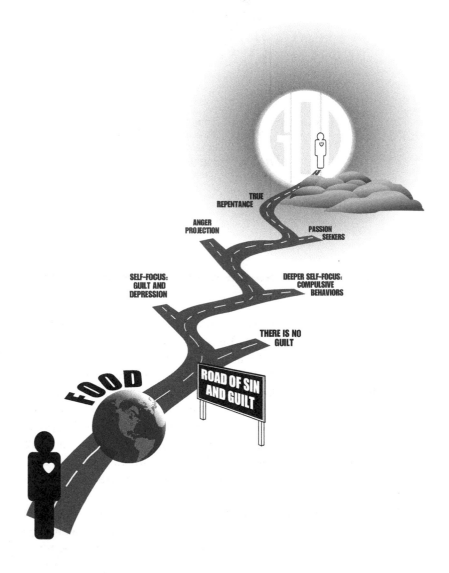

Figure 18-1: Focusing on the world inevitably will lead us to sin, which causes us to feel the pain of guilt. Five dead-end paths offer false hope of escaping the path of sin and guilt, but we can genuinely escape that path only through true repentance that leads to God.

unmerciful, jealous, untrusting, angry, moody, self-righteous, and they are regular party-poopers. What a damper the older brother put on the fatted calf banquet party for the repentant younger brother (Luke 15). Both manifestations are equally wrong. Even though one manifestation of a crooked heart seems more visible than the other, be sure that the unrepentant heart will come forth. "A good tree cannot bear bad fruit and a bad tree cannot bear good fruit" (Matthew 7:18). The good heart emptied and refilled with the character and loving nature of the Father will be both loving and outwardly self-controlled.

If the mind and heart continue down their own unrepentant path (you continue to overeat, binge, etc.), the path of sin, guilt, depression, and anger is inevitable. We are at a crossroad. As long as we do not repent, we will stay in the guilty state—and it is painful. This pain was meant to urge us to repent. Unfortunately, many times our own hearts, or even well-meaning counselors, have encouraged us to take one or more of these wrong paths discussed in the upcoming pages. These paths are obviously dead-end streets of destructive cycles.

Some advisors have given good, strong counsel that leads to repentance. However, since there are increasing numbers of depressed, obese people, we conclude that these wise teachers are in the minority. We are to blame as much as the counselors. We are the ones who went looking for advice that would lead us to a pill to numb the guilt, or that would tell us to do just about anything except to eat less food or repent from focusing on self. We would much rather sit in a small group year after year and justify the reasons we have not changed.

There is only one path to take to get rid of the guilty feeling—the path of true repentance that leads to God. The principles of the Weigh Down Workshop[t] are helping thousands upon thousands to take the path to true repentance. This chapter is hopefully an eye opener to expose the five deceptive paths that are freshly paved and that lure us in—in hopes that we can put off or avoid true repentance. No matter who is to blame, let us expose these dead-end paths so that we can turn around, get off them, and get back on the right path.

Dead-end path—"There is no guilt"

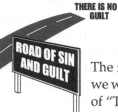

The first wrong path that we will expose is the path of "There Is No Guilt." This is more like an expressway than a path, because it is taken by many people both inside and outside the church. Most overweight people report that they are in a persistent state of feeling guilty and depressed, and that fatigue often accompanies these feelings. The feelings are often intertwined; the person cannot remember what started the destructive cycle. Did the overeating lead to guilt, or did the depression lead to overeating?

Obviously, there are differing schools of thought and much confusion. We know deep down that we feel bad or have a heaviness in the heart if we keep bowing down to the idol of food, yelling at our spouse and children, controlling our family, depending on drugs, or repeating secret sins. Is this heavy guilt-depression feeling legitimate, or is it a counterfeit feeling from Satan, the accuser? Should we ignore it or claim, as some theologians suggest, that guilt is no longer an issue once you believe in Jesus, since He died for our sins? Some preachers/pastors believe it is blasphemous or insulting to say that people need to worry about sin or disobedience after they have been rescued from Egypt. But look at this scripture from Hebrews 3:7–4:1.

So, as the Holy Spirit says: "Today, if you hear his voice, do not harden your hearts as you did in the rebellion, during the time of testing in the desert, where your fathers tested and tried me and for forty years saw what I did. That is why I was angry with that generation, and I said, 'Their hearts are always going astray, and they have not known my ways.' So I declared on oath in my anger, 'They shall never enter my rest.'" See to it, brothers, that none of you has a sinful, unbelieving heart that turns away from the living God. But encourage one another daily, as long as it is called Today, so that none of you may be hardened by sin's deceitfulness. We have come to share in Christ if we hold firmly till the end the confidence we had at first. As has just been said: "Today, if you hear his voice, do not harden your hearts as you did in the rebellion." Who were they who heard and rebelled? Were they not all those Moses led out of Egypt? And with whom was he angry for forty years? Was it not with those who sinned, whose bodies fell in the desert? And to whom did God swear that they would never enter his rest if not to those who disobeyed? So we see that they were not able to enter, because of their unbelief. Therefore, since the promise of entering his rest still stands, let us be careful that none of you be found to have fallen short of it.

So, our hearts tell us something is wrong as we sit on the church pew week after week wrapped and clothed in the same destructive behaviors that we have had all these years. How then should we handle these guilty feelings?

One thing we can agree on is that we do not want this guilt-depressed feeling around. The guilt feeling is real. It is not from Satan. He is not in the business of making us feel guilty if we have shunned God by bowing down to the refrigerator. Satan wants us to believe that it is OK to keep running to the box of chocolates for comfort. Rather, it is God who has programmed our conscience to make us feel guilty when we do wrong, since wrongdoing leads to death of a heart of love for Him. Look at this scripture in Romans 6:16: "Don't you know that when you offer yourselves to someone to obey him as slaves, you are slaves to the one whom you obey—whether you are slaves to sin, which leads to death, or to obedience, which leads to righteousness?"

God gets our attention when our flame of love for Him is being blown out, and He fans the flame of love for Him by rewarding us when we do right, traveling the path of love to Him—a road to life! If you only have a flickering flame, or even if you are only a smoldering wick, do not fret. Jesus showed God's love by loving the most unlovable individuals—even people who had murdered Christians—such as the Apostle Paul. Isaiah 42:3 refers to Jesus, and this passage is repeated in Matthew 12:20: "A bruised reed he will not break, and a smoldering wick he will not snuff out . . . ." Just as you are careful not to smother a smoldering stick so that you can get the fire blazing eventually, God or Jesus would never do anything to put out the small, smoldering piece of love in your heart.

It is true that you cannot do works and get away with disguising the *absence* of love in your heart. Attempting to camouflage your heart will not get you into His presence. Do you want a marriage partner who does things around you and for you, but who does not genuinely care for you? Of course not! God is no different.

Works will not hide an unloving heart. What about halfway loving God—is that OK? Should you continue loving your worldly lovers while God is madly in love with you? In other words, should you continue in sin that grace may abound? "By no means!" Romans 6:2 says. God has gotten down on His knees (so to speak) to propose to you. Especially if you consider that He sacrificed His only Son for your hand in marriage or this covenant relationship. I liken grace to this proposal picture. How can we turn this down? And if we accept, how could we run after another lover? This proposal from God demands a response of wholehearted love and faith from us. Remember, Scripture tells us that to God, "The only thing that counts is faith expressing itself through love" (Galatians 5:6b).

Bottom line: when we catch ourselves being faithful to the refrigerator instead of Him, it is like being caught in the act of adultery. We cannot love two masters. We feel guilty when God catches us adoring something besides Him. Would you expect your spouse to allow you to love another? Then how do we expect the Father to? All throughout the Old and New Testaments, God gets upset at His children for even turning to another lover (idol), much less trying to talk Him into letting all three get into the same bed. That has always been our problem—we want it both ways.

Many will beg God to please love them but let them keep their other loves too! If we continue in a sinful behavior, we will eventually become calloused and have no more guilty feelings because our conscience has been seared, which is a frightening thought. See Ephesians 4:17–27 and 1 Timothy 4:2.

Take it from me, you do not want it both ways—you will be miserable. Titus 2:11–14 says, "For the grace of God that brings salvation has appeared to all men. It teaches us to say 'No' to ungodliness and worldly passions, and to live self-controlled, upright and godly lives in this present age, while we wait for the blessed hope —the glorious appearing of our great God and Savior, Jesus Christ, who gave himself for us to redeem us from all wickedness and to purify for himself a people that are his very own, eager to do what is good."

Jesus redeemed us and set us apart to love the Father. The word *holy* means "set apart." And this group is *eager* to do that.

Passage after passage in the Old and New Testaments cries out the message that we are not to continue in sin (giving our hearts to something other than God). Again in Colossians 3:5–8,12–14, you see the repentance language: *"Put to death,* therefore, whatever belongs to your earthly nature: sexual immorality, impurity, lust, evil desires and greed, which is idolatry. Because of these, the wrath of God is coming. You used to walk in these ways, in the life you once lived. But now you must *rid yourselves* of all such things as these: anger, rage, malice, slander, and filthy language from your lips . . . Therefore, as God's chosen people, holy and dearly loved, *clothe yourselves* with compassion, kindness, humility, gentleness and patience. Bear with each other and forgive whatever grievances you may have against one another. Forgive as the LORD forgave you. And over all these virtues *put on love,* which binds them all together in perfect unity."

When you find this grace, accept it, and receive it, you will have a response of love in your heart which will be revealed in your actions. Notice this scripture passage uses verbs that are all active verbs, not passive verbs. Those actions will not be *work*—if you love Him. If you do not, it will be work, and He does not even want to see it. It is easy if you love Him! I liken it to a chemical reaction, with Jesus' love and sacrifice being the catalyst that makes this happen.

If we are not careful, we could end up joining the masses both inside and outside the church building who believe there is no guilt. They either do not want to or do not know they are to accept this proposal of a relationship—or as the Bible states, "put off," "put to death," "rid yourselves," "clothe yourselves," "put on love,"—or say no to the old way of love of the world. They repeat the same sin over and over. They keep giving their heart to their other lover.

Woe to the Bible teachers or church leaders who continue to paint a picture of God as a nonpassionate, unresponsive sissy. Woe to those who claim that the blood of Jesus was sacrificed to allow God's children to have two lovers!

Unfortunately, I know people whose pastor or preacher has made them feel guilty for admitting that they do not feel right before God! In other words, he made them feel guilty for admitting they are guilty. They should have been encouraged to turn their heart toward home. Guilt would disappear and acceptance pour in.

So, yes, there *is* guilt when we do not correctly respond to this grace. It is a painful reminder that we are on the wrong path. Following the path of the ultimate deceit, "There is no guilt," will get you nowhere. Get off of this highway now.

No matter the number of diets you have tried, or even if you weigh 600 pounds or more—your past does not stop you from turning your heart to God right now, drinking deeply from the spring of living water, and finding abundant life. No longer should we continue overeating because we think it is okay with God. Jesus came to forgive your sins, and then He calls you to repent of your old loves and to "marry" yourself to the Father. True repentance is foundational.

Dead-end path—Self-focus/guilt-depression

The second path is different from the first one. The first path is a belief that there is no guilt. Its travelers usually surround themselves with people who adopt "I'm OK, you're OK" attitudes to justify their indulgences.

This second path, the highway of depression, is one that is well traveled. Travelers on this highway do not know how to turn, or even that they can turn. These travelers are not calloused over; rather, they feel the guilt that God has sent. However, they have been trying to change everything and everybody else and not themselves, so they remain in a continual state of what I call *guilt-depression*.

To get off the broad highway of *guilt-depression* and onto the narrow path of joy and peace, we must find the origin of *guilt-depres-*

sion. To start, let us look at the first few words from Genesis 4:2b–8:
Now Abel kept flocks, and Cain worked the soil. In the course of
time Cain brought some of the fruits of the soil as an offering to
the LORD. But Abel brought fat portions from some of the first-
born of his flock. The LORD looked with favor on Abel and his
offering, but on Cain and his offering he did not look with favor.
So Cain was very angry, and his face was downcast.

Then the LORD said to Cain, "Why are you angry? Why is your
face downcast? If you do what is right, will you not be accepted?
But if you do not do what is right, sin is crouching at your door;
it desires to have you, but you must master it."

Now Cain said to his brother Abel, "Let's go out to the field."
And while they were in the field, Cain attacked his brother Abel
and killed him.

Guilt-depression

First we learn from this passage on Cain and Abel that anger and
depression (downcast feeling) accompanied the first sin and every
sin thereafter. These feelings are normal and were programmed into
us by God. Everyone has
sinned, so all people have felt
this *guilt-depression* that we are
referring to in varying degrees.
This passage holds so many
answers to deliverance from
depression and anger. For
one, we see that if you

sin without repenting, you automatically feel angry and downcast or depressed. God is really trying to get our attention to make us turn around off this dead-end street and turn down the narrow path of true repentance. If we stick our finger in the fire once, most of us will not do it again. We can learn. But, unfortunately, as bad as the guilt and depression feel, the substitute sympathy it brings feels even better—temporarily, that is. After the self-focus and self-pity feelings have run their course, we are left with the real underneath feeling of guilt, depression, rejection, isolation, and loneliness.

You can find people who will tell you feeling depressed is an illness and out of your control. But just as quickly as depression comes from sin, joy comes from repentance. We have seen hundreds walk out of depression who were previously diagnosed as "clinical," implying a physiological abnormality. These people accomplished this—not by embracing the medicine cabinet, but rather, wholeheartedly embracing the will of God. There are indeed rare cases of all kinds of physical abnormalities, but they are just that—rare.

The truth will set you free

This is hard teaching. The nearer that Jesus got to the cross, the fewer the people that followed Him. Many of His teachings were hard, and once His disciples said, " 'This is a hard teaching. Who can accept it?' Aware that his disciples were grumbling about this, Jesus said to them, 'Does this offend you? . . . The Spirit gives life; the flesh counts for nothing. The words I have spoken to you are spirit and they are life' " (John 6:60b–63). It is hard to swallow that self-pity, and self-focus, and our own sin are all choice, but they are. God did not send Cain to group therapy class to discuss and justify why he was depressed. He gave him no counterfeit acceptance—rather, He gave him advice to repent and get it right the next time. He loved him enough to give him that truth!

Perhaps guilt-depression has been so misdiagnosed because well-meaning counselors have been afraid to tell hurting people the truth. Perhaps they would lose a client, or, more than likely, the truth is not outlined in the latest psychology book.

But once again, I look at the fruit. I see the masses who, liberated by God's truths that they learn in the Weigh Down Workshop[t], are no longer depressed and no longer on pills. Have we forgotten the fact that when you tell people the truth, the truth will set them free (John 8:32)? Can you imagine a surgeon refusing to cut on his patient if surgery is required to save the patient's life? The surgeon must cut the body open to remove the cancer. It might hurt the depressed person to tell the truth to remove the infirmity. But look at this scripture: "For the word of God is living and active. Sharper than any double-edged sword, it penetrates even to dividing soul and spirit, joints and marrow; it judges the thoughts and attitudes of the heart. Nothing in all creation is hidden from God's sight. Everything is uncovered and laid bare before the eyes of him to whom we must give account" (Hebrews 4:12–13).

The truth is like a knife, but the lie or misdiagnosis makes the depression chronic and more miserable.

This guilt-depression we are referring to does not have its roots in the physiological, such as the down time experienced by women a few hours before menstruation. Nor is it godly sorrow that even the sinless Jesus experienced, but rather, it is a feeling that has its roots in wanting to keep food as a first love and God's approval at the same time. God wanted Cain to give up his firstfruits—but Cain was sorry and angry and depressed. There is a difference between godly sorrow and worldly sorrow. "Even if I caused you sorrow by my letter, I do not regret it. Though I did regret it —I see that my letter hurt you, but only for a little while — yet now I am happy, not because you were made sorry, but because your sorrow led you to repentance. For you became sorrowful as God intended and so were not harmed in any way by us. Godly sorrow brings repentance that leads to salvation and leaves no regret, but worldly sorrow brings death. See what this godly sorrow has produced in you: what earnestness, what eagerness to clear yourselves, what indignation, what alarm, what longing, what concern, what readiness to see justice done" (2 Corinthians 7:8–11a).

We get angry at God when we cannot have our food and be thin, too! We get angry when God won't change His laws to let us have acceptance and the love of food at the same time. We are trying hard to control God and change His laws, and we need desperately to control our own greed and love His laws.

Peace and joy are the results of godly sorrow and true repentance because the acceptance of God floods the soul. Even your countenance will change. Notice how easy it is to make this connection we are talking about. Make it a point to observe how depressed you feel when you mess up and how great you feel when you obey God and eat right and lose weight. You can master this!

Dysfunctional families and abused lives

Again referring to the Cain and Abel passage, you can see that we learn many things. As we have discussed before, the world's first family was dysfunctional: Cain killed his brother with a rock! Any sin in a family member affects the other family members. All have sinned, therefore all families are dysfunctional. We must no longer continue to let the label "dysfunctional" serve as an excuse for our behavior.

There is more. It has always run counter to my advice for people to continue to talk about, dwell on, or in any way use history to excuse their present behavior. In other words, it is not logical to believe that a person's having been molested in childhood is why they are continuing to adore the indulgence of food. I do not see the connection; however, I do see the "excuse," just as I see the excuse of "I am afraid to get thin because men may notice me." These people just do not want to let go of the food, for they love that relationship with food more than the relationship with men or God. It is a choice. If you have some special history, genetic makeup, dysfunctional family, or critical event that *makes* you cling to the refrigerator—I have not seen it. We cling because we love it.

Weigh Down Workshop[†] participants who refused to dwell in the past and who stayed in the present are the ones who ate less food and lost weight! Almost everyone coming to Weigh Down Workshop[†] had previously been counseled into spending hours resurrecting dysfunctional ancestry. Many wanted to tell me that they had just learned through counselling that a family member had sexually abused them, and that is why they were overweight! My advice would be the same every time, regardless of whether this revelation about their past turned out to be true. Look at the Apostle Paul. What a horrible history he could have dwelled on. He put to death innocent people—not only that, God's innocent children! He imprisoned many, and those prisons were not your big screen TV, basketball court, Basic Four food group facilities back then. The Apostle Paul never dwelled on all his murders—never talked about them, but just briefly reflected on the past and acknowledged that he had been the "chiefest of sinners." He did not describe the details or bring up all the emotions from the past. He simply talked about the saving grace and forgiveness of Jesus Christ. He moved the subject "off" himself and talked about the present or the future—never self-focused stories of the past. Now, if that is how the Apostle Paul took care of a horrible history that could have haunted him, then let us please allow history to rest—especially if God has erased it from your memory banks!

I see people—at the request of their own counselors—make major deals out of apologizing to people who did not know they had even been wronged or they confront people who had wronged them when they were thirteen years old (twenty-five years ago). And yet they had not repented of their own sin. What a mess!

Jesus did not say to the adulterous woman, "Go and fix everything and everyone you have wronged." No! He just said go and "you" sin no more. Here's the point: one is a focus on other people and their sins, and one is a focus on your own sins and your own relationship with God. Your own reconciliation with God is the goal.

A God-focused relationship will automatically result in a better relationship with mankind. As you just focus on laying down your own strongholds, you will become merciful because you see the degree of difficulty. A forgiving nature is birthed in the heart of a truly repentant person. Once you have truly repented and turned, God may lead you to restore relationships. The repentant tax collector offered to go back and pay people he had wronged. But, for the most part, sinners were not asked to look back. Here is what John the Baptist told sinners: " 'What should we do then?' the crowd asked. John answered, 'The man with two tunics should share with him who has none, and the one who has food should do the same.' Tax collectors also came to be baptized. 'Teacher,' they asked, 'what should we do?' 'Don't collect any more than you are required to,' he told them. Then some soldiers asked him, 'And what should we do?' He replied, 'Don't extort money and don't accuse people falsely —be content with your pay' " (Luke 3:10–14). They were asked to start that day being different.

These people were focused on having hurt the Father. If we are the victim, we need to know that everything that happens to us is screened by the Father.

My guess is that all of us have played both victim and abuser roles at some point in time. Whether you are the victim or abuser, repent of your own past and present sins. Reconciliation with God first and mankind second will be inevitable—not vice versa. God takes care of victims. Fear for the hearts of the abusers and pray for them, because this God of ours will take revenge on those who wrong us. He loves justice.

Turning depression around

In conclusion, guilt-depression is real. Self-pity, however, is not the way off this path. Self-pity is a feeling you are looking for, and it feels so good (we think) to feel sorry for self. For those who want out, you can repent and ask God to remove this depressed feeling. Hang on to Him hour by hour, and you will make it out of this black hole.

The response to this information can go two ways. You can either turn to God, make the choice not to go down the path of depression, and become healed, or you can take the path of :"She couldn't possibly understand what I have been through, so what can she tell me!" The second path is the "I want to feel sorry for myself again" path.

The person who is making the choice to enjoy the feeling of focus on self and self-pity, with the combination of the food binge and antidepressant, is just that—making the choice and loving the feeling. It just feels good to have a pity party and to be angry at someone else and medicate yourself with food and drugs. For some, it feels legal to move into a world of "no responsibility" as you lie on the bed until noon everyday. This is an untruth, of course! Again, looking for a feeling is not wrong—but you must go to God, for He is the one who can give you the fulfilled feeling you are looking for, with no guilty side effects and no physical side effects—except good ones.

The conversation or thought process of many of the people who want to make the choice of depression is predictable. They want to think that others could get out of depression, but not them. They put themselves in a category that cannot repent, for "others have not had as hard a life as I have."

I have talked to many depressed people, and I have noticed a pattern of excuses for those who do not want to let go of depression. "Happiness, good things, and nice clothes are all for someone else, not me. I am a loser. My background is worse than others'. I am a failure at working places. I feel like I have messed up so much. I am never worthy of any blessings. I rarely feel like anyone would want to meet me or care about what I think. When I think about it, I have never pleased my spouse or children. My father or mother never told me I did a good job, or they have never said that they are proud of me. I don't want to get out of the house, and I don't know if I have enough fight in me to get out of depression. I feel very unimportant."

Most people caught up in this cycle of depression feel that the circumstance is what is to blame for the depression. "My depression is from work ending, or from doing work I do not like because people at work are taking advantage of me. My depression is from an unfulfilled home life or from someone not liking me . . . I feel like I have been forgotten."

Yes, some people have more problems than others. But if depression was circumstantial, then there should have been more depressed people during The Great Depression in the 1930s, but there were not. People were very poor and hardly ever got meat to eat or shoes to wear. These circumstances did not propagate more crime nor depression from the individuals. The book *The Hiding Place* is the famous story of Corrie Ten Boom and her sister Betsie, who lived for one year in a Nazi concentration camp. Betsie found good even in the plague of fleas in their bunks. She noticed that the guards would leave them alone at night due to the fleas. She knew it was from God, for it provided them with a window of time to share the Bible with the other prisoners. She never lost sight that God was with her, even under the torture of that hellish situation. Betsie's dying words were, "Corrie, we have got to go back and tell them that there is no pit so deep that Jesus is not still deeper. They will listen to us, because we have been there."* Betsie focused on God and His working around her and let God take care of her. Her outside body died, but the inside of her was the carving of a soul more beautiful than the Hope diamond.

People may think that the etiology of depression is circumstantial. Most of the depressed people I have talked to felt that depression was mostly caused by circumstances wherein people did not approve of them. They never feel good enough, pretty enough, smart enough. All of this is a horizontal focus on man and not a vertical focus on God. It is all a focus on a comparison of self to other people and to their standards. This person's stronghold or idol is approval of men. This person's false God is in looking for fulfillment in other people—not God.

God will not let your idols feed you, and this person will never get the approval of man until they lay it down and not desire it anymore. In other words, if you want and seek the approval of God first—He will give you back the approval of man. That is something only God can give, and He can take it away. You cannot obtain it with your power!

If this seems to describe you, the next step is to figure out how to let go of that stronghold. Going to God is the answer. Go back and read the "Rise Above" and "Stay Awake" chapters. If you are focusing on God, you do not have time to focus on yourself. Focusing on self and the approval of man is a sin. By calling on God's help, you can end the desire for the food, drugs, and the approval of man. This scripture in Proverbs points this out: "Fear of man will prove to be a snare, but whoever trusts in the LORD is kept safe" (Proverbs 29:25).

Do not expect depression to end if you give up just one of your idols. You may say that you have given up the approval of man and

---

* Corrie Ten Boom, *The Hiding Place*, Inspirational Press, New York, 1983. Page 171.

yet you still do not feel good, so you stay on your antidepressants. My question to you is: have you lost your weight yet? Well, do not expect for God to remove the guilt-depression until you do. Then you may be able to give up your antidepressants, too. God will sustain you hour by hour as you choose to give these crutches up hour by hour. After years of overeating or overdosing, you *might* experience some adjustment physiologically and emotionally. Stay on your knees in prayer, and God will lift you up!

Ultimately, if we continue looking for every excuse—we need to face the fact that we do not want to give up our idol of food or depression.

Dead-end path—Deeper self-focus/deeper depression

Demon possession

I want to briefly mention some behaviors that may result from demon possession. I do not believe in the practice of going into every room in a house and casting out demons. Neither Jesus nor his disciples cast demons out of people's rooms. Jesus said "The reason the Son of God appeared was to destroy the devil's work" (1 John 3:8b). I believe Him on this

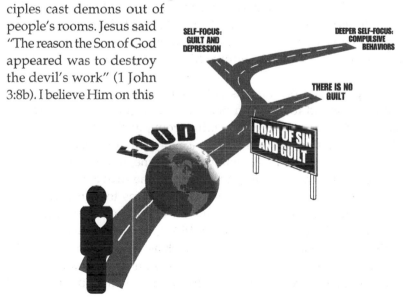

issue. Satan has falsely accused God and characterized Him as a being that you would not want a relationship with. Jesus has destroyed that evil work. God is the One you want to get in good with. At this point in time, I believe that there is a difference between idolatry and demon possession and, therefore, these are handled differently.

My experience tells me most of our problems stem from idolatry, a decision to give the heart to something on this earth. The origin of this evil is from our own evil desire. "When tempted, no one should say, 'God is tempting me.' For God cannot be tempted by evil, nor does he tempt anyone; but each one is tempted when, by his own evil desire, he is dragged away and enticed. Then, after desire has conceived, it gives birth to sin; and sin, when it is full-grown, gives birth to death" (James 1:13–15).

Possession by an evil spirit is talked about all over the Bible. In the Old Testament, the boy David would play and sing psalms, and it would drive the evil spirits away from King Saul. In the New Testament, Jesus and His disciples drove out demons. But from what I can see, in almost every case, the demon-possessed person was brought to Jesus rather than the person approaching Jesus. One exception where the demoniac approached Jesus is the account of Legion, found in Mark 5:2–20 and Luke 8:26–39. These demon-possessed people were described in the following ways: "It scarcely ever leaves him . . ." and ". . . throws him into convulsions . . ." (Luke 9:39).

The possessed person was not asked to do anything or to have faith or respond to "Do you believe?" type questions by Jesus, as happened in cases involving healing from physical ailments or forgiveness of sin. After Jesus spoke a word, the demons, subject to Him, would come out. "When evening came, many who were demon-possessed were brought to him, and he drove out the spirits with a word and healed all the sick. This was to fulfill what was spoken through the prophet Isaiah: 'He took up our infirmities and carried our diseases' " (Matthew 8:16,17). The person was restored with no additional commandment, such as "go and sin no more."

Perhaps the scourge of demon possession is not from our own evil desires (such as idolatry), but from leaving an empty heart that is not devoted to anything—especially to God. Satan gets a foothold and enters. Biblical accounts indicate that young people were a target, as young, impressionable people are more prone to have this "open book" type of a heart. And, of course, the Gospel of Matthew warns "When an evil spirit comes out of a man, it goes through arid places seeking rest and does not find it. Then it says, 'I will return to the house I left.' When it arrives, it finds the house unoccupied, swept clean and put in order. Then it goes and takes with it seven other spirits more wicked than itself, and they go in and live there. And the final condition of that man is worse than the first" (Matthew 12:43–45a).

This type of topic usually scares us if we feel like it is something that is out of our control. But do not fear. I have found that if you suspect demon possession in yourself or in a loved one, the thing to do is get down on your knees and bring yourself or the person you love to the feet of Jesus in your prayer. Jesus healed and still heals many. We will never get to sing enough praises to Jesus Christ the Savior.

So what Jesus' followers found out was that "even the demons submit to us in your name." Jesus replied, "I saw Satan fall like lightning from heaven. I have given you authority to trample on snakes and scorpions and to overcome all the power of the enemy; nothing will harm you" (Luke 10:17b–19). God is in control of every little thing.

Deeper guilt-depression

However, if you remain on the path of idolatry and the sin is not reversed, this separation from God or this feeling of hopeless isolation can lead us into deeper depression and into some equally bizarre behaviors and major mood swings, due in part to the highs and lows of antidepressants. Continued unaddressed sin will result in an inability to concentrate, decreased activity level, restlessness and sleep disturbance.

The Mayo Clinic Family Health reports that more than 1.5 million people take tranquilizers on a regular basis. They also report that people who take them more than four months in a row may become addicted.** Look at this passage from the Psalms by King David when he sinned: "O Lord, do not rebuke me in your anger or discipline me in your wrath. For your arrows have pierced me, and your hand has come down upon me. Because of your wrath there is no health in my body; my bones have no soundness because of my sin. My guilt has overwhelmed me like a burden too heavy to bear. My wounds fester and are loathsome because of my sinful folly. I am bowed down and brought very low; all day long I go about mourning. My back is filled with searing pain; there is no health in my body. I am feeble and utterly crushed; I groan in anguish of heart . . . For I am about to fall, and my pain is ever with me. I confess my iniquity; I am troubled by my sin" (Psalm 38:1–8,17,18).

Coping paths

Continued sin can lead you into deeper isolation from God, and the needy person may resort to many things in an attempt to "make it" in life without the foundational and structural walls that God provides. This person might try to cope by grasping at a counterfeit attention or acceptance—people's attention and acceptance.

Efforts to get attention and approval from people (the counterfeit of true acceptance from God) can manifest themselves in many ways. For example, anorexia nervosa is a condition wherein the person refuses to eat as the body calls for food so that the person becomes extraordinarily thin. This behavior is successful in drawing attention; however, the anorexic person needs to know that this behavior will not be rewarded by God with the acceptance that is needed. This means of control does not bear fruit. Wake up—have you "made" your life better? No, but He can. Obey Him with your eating. Then go to Him with your needs.

One route that frequently reveals the lust-focused heart is the path of compulsive behaviors, which include "nervous habits." These vary in degree and are, in some cases, severe. Examples include nail bit-

---

** Mayo Foundation for Medical Education and Research, *Mayo Clinic Family Health*. Rochester, Minn.: IVI Publishing Inc., 1996.

ing, hair pulling, thumb sucking, and picking at the skin to the point of making sores. These are outward manifestations of a heart in turmoil, one lacking the peace and trust of the Spirit of God, a heart focused on self. I have seen nail biting to the point that it drew blood, hair pulling that resulted in baldness, people with persistent scabs on their skin from constant picking, and grown adults still sucking their thumbs. Self-mutilating people, who claw at or hurt themselves to get attention, may ultimately go so far as to attempt or achieve suicide. It is not God's will for us to be so enslaved; His goal is to be our Savior, to free us from enslaving behaviors.

Many people are extremely needy. Some migrate permanently toward psychiatrists, psychologists, clinics, or doctors for help to alleviate the pain in their lives—but to no avail. Sometimes these people do not know that they are looking for attention or sympathy from mankind, but what they really need is acceptance from God.

People with self-focused behaviors know that something is wrong, but they keep looking for physical diagnoses. If these people get enough MRIs or make enough doctor appointments, they can get someone to find something wrong with them. It is amazing how quickly an unsupportive family (the ones at home who have a hard time feeling sorry for your overweight condition when they see you binge every night at 10 o'clock) becomes supportive when shown a diagnosis that helps "justify" overeating or any mood swings. The now sympathetic family, impressed by the long, technical-sounding diagnosis and the prescribed pills, is persuaded the person has a physiological problem, that he is legitimately, clinically, and chronically unfortunate. This path is expensive, and it still does not achieve what the person really needs—acceptance that starts with repentance of the wrong behavior. The counterfeit—sympathy—will not fill up the hurting heart.

These people do definitely have something wrong in their lives— they are not hypochondriacs. It is just that they have been looking for diagnoses and cures at hospitals that address physical conditions, while what they really need is more readily found at church.

Self-focused phobias

Another area of concern is that this feeling of hopeless isolation can play on phobias and spawn all kinds of self-focused fears. People who feel a lack of acceptance from God, as Cain felt, also fear that others do not accept or like them. This fear can manifest itself in paranoia and panic attacks, agoraphobia, self-mutilation, suicidal tendencies, and mania (feeling very "high") and then depression (feeling very "low"). This manic-depressive mood swing behavior is eventually aggravated by the highs and lows caused by antidepressants and prescribed pills. Patients will take uppers and clean the house or rake the yard until two o'clock in the morning (high). Now they want sleeping pills to go to sleep. This is not a good pattern to become dependent on. The side effects are due to medication—not some genetic, chronic problem. In other words, the uppers give the person a burst of energy until they are "spent," only adding to the unbalanced lifestyle. The solution is to stop depending on the medicine cabinet for good feelings and for energy or for sleep. God can give both without costly side effects, ". . . for he grants sleep to those he loves" (Psalm 127:2).

Sin-laden people experience an "out of control" feeling. Nothing seems to go right, and the harder they try to "control," the worse the environment gets. These people have not experienced giving their heart over to God to the point that they can ask what they want and it will be done! If they have not experienced frequently answered prayers, then no wonder they feel "out of control." Answered prayers are given to those whose hearts are "abiding" in Jesus. "Dear friends, if our hearts do not condemn us, we have confidence before God and receive from him anything we ask, because we obey his commands and do what pleases him" (1 John 3:21,22). I could write a whole book on examples of answered prayers; not that every prayer results in people getting what they pray for, but there is a definite correlation between answered prayer and wholehearted obedience to God. Just as you seem to have more cooperation from your spouse when you have put his or her needs first, it is true with God also. It is just common sense.

Sin-laden people have not experienced going to God for everything, so they feel they have no control over their environment, and some try to cope by making their world smaller and smaller. If thrust outside their environment, they might have panic attacks. To cope, they collapse their world down so small, in an attempt to keep it a manageable size, that they confine themselves to their houses. Eventually, some go so far as to feel safe only within the confines of their own bedrooms. Many spend hours worrying about their safety. Sometimes it manifests itself in "germ" phobia, which is rooted in fear for self and an attempt to "control" the environment. This can lead to some obsessive-compulsive cleaning behaviors. It can also lead to obsessive-compulsive purification of the inside of the body, resulting in weekly colon cleansing with combinations of laxatives. This is potentially damaging to the gut or large intestine. *Sympathy is no substitute for acceptance or comfort from God.*

Sometimes people on this path can become so self-focused that they cannot seem to go more than a few minutes without returning to their self-absorption. A hurting heart on this path might try manic behaviors, then switch to depressed behaviors for sympathy. Sympathy feels good for a while, but it leaves people feeling like a baby and leaves them feeling pretty empty. Sympathy is no substitute for acceptance or comfort from God.

People on this path might become very talkative and loud, then get very, very quiet. They cry, then pout, then break out in rages. Anger is addressed on the next wrong path in this book. Sexually abused people often hang on to the story, for it always musters up repetitive sympathy and counterfeit justification of their overeating. To get God's acceptance, they need to know what God wants, and they need to do what God wants them to do. Self-focus can be reversed by repenting. Then the besetting sin can be repented of and the acceptance from God rushes through. Finally the self-focused disorders start to disappear. We have witnessed many people turn their hearts back to God, and He has erased their annoying panic attacks with a rush of confidence in Him. *The mind focuses upward—not inward!* Controllers start letting God be the God.

Chronic anxiety

Some people have not known what to do with life on this earth—much less the guilt. They have gotten caught up in a path of chronic anxiety. It is like a friend. They look for something to worry about. They worry about things that may or may not be real. They worry about the past, present and the future. They worry about things that will never happen. If you were to take a survey of these worriers, you would find that only a small number of them have legitimate concerns. They are anxious about their life, and if that does not give them enough to chew on, they will worry about their neighbor's business. They keep things stirred up. Peace is not in their vocabulary. To take their focus off of self is almost impossible—it is their stronghold.

The anxiety-ridden highway is the one most traveled and has funded several multi-billion-dollar industries in this country. Tobacco, wine, beer, hard liquor, tranquilizers, and antidepressants are being sold by the truckloads. We use these substances to numb ourselves, and then we give them to our children. Not only has the over-abuse drained our pocketbooks—it has left our physical bodies in bad shape.

Are we less anxious as a population? No! We have more anxiety than ever, and we have become slaves to substances. They do cover up the guilty feeling that we do not want to feel, yet the effect of the drink or drug eventually wears off, and we feel worse than before. Increasing the dosage is inevitable if we want the same effect. When we come back down off the substance, we see that we are farther behind on our projects at work, and the house is messier than it was before. We are more behind on our bills, and the family is more disappointed in us than they were even a few months ago. Anger runs even deeper. Many times, families are split by the wedge created by the use of a numbing agent. Our children suffer from this path we have chosen. When we see grown adults sucking their thumbs or biting their nails until they bleed, pulling their hair out for comfort, getting numbed with alcohol by mid-morning, or stuffing in even more food when they are already sixty-plus pounds overweight, we know the world is hurting, but these worldly substances are no match to the feelings of energy and comfort God can provide.

A very common manifestation of compulsive behavior is cigarette smoking. In spite of the research, I do not believe it is only the body that becomes addicted to the nicotine, but, also, the anxious spirit does. As we have discussed before, I believe the soul's addiction is stronger than the body's. The body is quite happy at the decrease of carbon monoxide down the lungs. But the ripping of the soul from the world affects body and soul. The withdrawals spiritually are hard to measure and vary from soul to soul.

If a person will redirect his focus from himself to God and allow God to help him rise above the temptations, then he can be set free from that stronghold. This is true not only of tobacco abuse, but also of alcohol and pills. Instead of the body being dependent on nicotine, it shows signs immediately that it loves any decrease or even quitting "cold turkey." I have never seen anyone die when they eat less food, smoke fewer cigarettes, drink significantly less alcohol, or take fewer antidepressants. However, I see the withdrawal being severe if this gap or void is not filled in with God. The withdrawal is the soul ripping itself away from the world. It hurts. Only the Savior can dissolve this kind of superglue.

How to "come down" off of addictive substances

Please do not misunderstand me on this point: to rise above the world you must simultaneously turn away from the world and toward God. Half-measures will leave you emptier and more depressed than if you had stayed firmly planted in the world.

Jesus once urged a wealthy young man to give away all he possessed *and* follow him. (See Luke 18.) He would never find completeness in his worldly possessions—only in Jesus. Sadly, the young man rejected Jesus' counsel; he could not bear to risk the lifestyle he already knew, even for a chance of filling up with Jesus. Can you imagine how he would have felt if he had followed only half of Jesus' advice, giving away all he had but then not following Jesus? With the comfort of neither his possessions nor of the Lord, he would have been absolutely miserable! Likewise, giving up antidepressants or the food and not replacing it with love of God might make you feel like what people call "crashing." You must depend on God and ask Him into your heart, and use all the principles that we have outlined in this book.

If you decide you are ready to give up your guilt-depression self-focus path which usually includes antidepressants, then remember: do not try to *just* give them up; give them up *and* at the same time replace them with a close, loving relationship with God. Otherwise, you might sink in the waters

General rules of letting go of any substance abuse:

1. No half-measures. Do not just give up pills; give them up *and* replace them with depending on God for the strength, "up feeling," and energy you believe the pills provide. If you are under heavy doses, stay under your doctor's care and have him provide a reasonable progression of decreasing the dependence on pills. Remember, when you let go of all your worthless idols, depression will end. " 'Those who cling to worthless idols forfeit the grace that could be theirs' " (Jonah 2:8). The depression is from clinging to the food, etc. So you need to give up the food. Your heart will be happy as you lose the weight, and the need for the pills will diminish.

2. Go to God for comfort. 2 Corinthians 1:3,4 says, "Praise be to the God and Father of our Lord Jesus Christ, the Father of compassion and the God of all comfort, who comforts us in all our troubles, so that we can comfort those in any trouble with the comfort we ourselves have received from God." God can give comfort better than anything or anyone. He may send someone your way, or you may receive an encouraging phone call or a positive scripture. Ask Him and He will comfort you. We people have an overwhelming need for comfort. We need to be calmed and assured. This is normal.

3. Make sure you ask God to guide you to God-focused counsel or small groups. So many groups will teach the opposite of Weigh Down^t and will only leave you in confusion. So many small groups try to make you dependent on them—not God.

Some try to make you lifelong members. People graduate from Weigh Down† classes all of the time. God can deliver you! Watch out for people who say "The answer is . . . ." For example, some say the "answer" is exercise. It may help, but it is not the answer. Do not get sidetracked on the voids—father void, mother void, or other labels. God is the answer. We have seen amazing breakthroughs of people coming out of bondage to depression drugs.

How to overcome fears

God is love. Whoever lives in love lives in God, and God in him. In this way, love is made complete among us so that we will have confidence on the day of judgment, because in this world we are like him. There is no fear in love. *But perfect love drives out fear, because fear has to do with punishment.* The one who fears is not made perfect in love. (1 John 4:16b–18)
I challenge all of us who feel trapped in fear to spend some time getting to know God. The Bible says that God wants us to have wisdom and understanding. He tells us to get to know Him, and when we get to know Him, we will love Him. Love of the Father gets rid of fear. Proverbs 3:21–26 assures us by saying, "My son, preserve sound judgment and discernment, do not let them out of your sight; they will be life for you, an ornament to grace your neck. Then you will go on your way in *safety*, and your foot will not stumble; when you lie down, you will not be afraid; when you lie down, your sleep will be sweet. Have no fear of sudden disaster or of the ruin that overtakes the wicked, for the LORD will be your confidence and will keep your foot from being snared."

If you experience panic attacks and the need to leave your house arises, approach it with prayer. Say, "God, I need to go to the grocery store today, and I am afraid of the crowds and the traffic. But, Lord, you are in control of everything that happens to me, and I will trust you. Give me strength." When you go to the store, go in faith that God will be with you. The next time, you will trust Him more readily, and even more the time after that. Soon you will be walking out the door in freedom and peace. No more panic attacks! The prescription drugs will not be your confidence, the small group will not be your confidence—the Lord will be your confidence!

For now, do not be afraid. Know this fact: call out to God and He will walk you through this. You will find yourself leaving the dependence on numbing agents, the compulsive behaviors, the self-focus, and the depression. With God's help, you can master this! Jesus left an ongoing sacrifice for all the mess-ups we have with our heart. Jesus came to show us how to become an Abel. And we long for it like a fish on the side of the bank longs for water.

Too often, physicians and counselors are just responding to what we demand—a simple diagnosis, a quick fix, and a pill to numb our pain. In fact, we doubt they are doing their job right if we walk out without a prescription! We must be brave enough to face the real problem and confess that the answer is found in seeking God *first*. If He wants us to use a physician or a counselor, God will direct us to one who will give us the counsel or treatment that God wants us to receive. Now, any substitute attention or band-aid therapy will be history!

Dead-end path—Anger, projection on others

This path is possibly chosen by people with pride. Their hearts may often be filled with unloving feelings—hate, murder, deception, uncontrolled rage, selfish ambition, and anger. They usually are manipulators, and they have learned how to control people. They are experts at projection, that is, blaming others for their problems. They decide their best defense is a good offense—attacking others! They try to rid themselves of their guilty feelings by getting angry and directing the anger, judgment, insults, and jabs at others. They go so far as to slander, sabotage, and lie about people. It is so much less painful to blame our behavior on those around us or even on God. The people who choose this path often cry out that they did not even ask to be on this earth—so they blame God for the pain of this guilt. But look closely again at these words from the first few pages of the Bible: "Then the LORD said to Cain, 'Why are you angry? Why is your face downcast? If you do what is right, will you not be accepted?' " (Genesis 4:6,7a).

The Cains of this world do not like people who are accepted by God if they, themselves, do not feel personally accepted by God. The Cain personalities would prefer to believe that people who claim to have a relationship with God are dreaming this up, confused, deluded, self-deceived, arrogant, bordering on blasphemous, and obviously in need of a crutch. They hate the word *favor*, and they really do not want to believe that God would actually favor someone. Since they have not experienced God's favor, they do not want anyone else to believe in it. They do not want to do what it takes to get favor, so once again they try to X this "favor" category out of life. They think that as long as they successfully mock the person who adores God and enjoys His acceptance, it might delay their having to submit their own hearts, minds, and souls to God. Anger to the point of murderous thoughts started with the first family unit and is still common today.

How many times has history repeated itself? Consider the accounts of people who were mistreated, tortured, imprisoned, or killed because they were visibly accepted by God on this earth: Abel murdered by Cain, Daniel thrown into the lion's den, Stephen stoned to death.

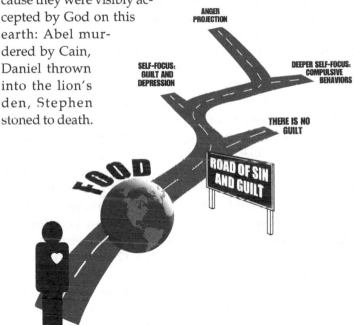

Chapters 37 through 50 of Genesis tell the story of the favored Joseph, a shepherd boy who was sold into slavery by his brothers.
Decades later, after Joseph had risen to the position of second-in-
command over all of Egypt, the guilt of what they had done to their
younger brother still haunted them.

Jealous, self-promoting men had the favored Jesus killed on a cross.
Getting rid of Jesus did not make them feel better, nor did Cain feel
better after killing Abel, the favored brother. What could Cain have
done to make himself feel better? God had the answer for him: not
"Get rid of the acceptable one and you will be promoted," but "If
you do what is right you will be accepted!"

There are modern-day Cains who would like to convince us
that God showed favor to the ones who are crazy about Him only
during biblical times. "God stopped showing personal favor two
thousand years ago. Right?" Wrong! He still today shows favor to
those who pursue righteousness. You can tell that He does in many
ways.

People attempt the "Cain solution" in the workplace daily. They
try to sabotage the boss's pet to "get ahead" or get themselves in
good with the boss. I have good news for those engaging in this
behavior. You can reverse course. You no longer have to go down
this rotten path of projection to get rid of your guilt feeling!

The problem that lies at the origin of this path is that the person
does not want to give their firstfruits to the Heavenly Father. You do
not mind taking this love from the Father, and you do not mind
giving Him a portion of your money, your Sunday morning, and a
whole list of things you like to give that come naturally. For example,
you like the command to go to church because you personally love
the fellowship. However, when He asks for what goes against your
will—for instance, your food—well, you are not so sure about that.
No one told you God was going to ask you to show your love for
Him by giving up the firstfruits (your other lovers). We do not like
handing over our lifelong idols. 1 John 2:15–17 says: "Do not love
the world or anything in the world. If anyone loves the world, the
love of the Father is not in him. For everything in the world —the
cravings of sinful man, the lust of his eyes and the boasting of what
he has and does —comes not from the Father but from the world.

The world and its desires pass away, but the man who does the will of God lives forever."

Again, we do not easily give up the one worldly stronghold He asks for, just as many married people do not easily give their spouses the main thing they want. They will give nice, decent things, but not the one or two things their spouses really desire. How you deal with the firstfruits will affect your stronghold, and ultimately, your relationships with God, your spouse, and your family. Many times, what God and your spouse want you to give up, are the very same strongholds.

Cain, not Abel, had this problem. Both brothers offered sacrifices of the work of their hands. Their outward behaviors were the same. Man may have a hard time seeing why God accepted one gift but not the other gift. You cannot tell by looking.

> Now Abel kept flocks, and Cain worked the soil. In the course of time Cain brought some of the fruits of the soil as an offering to the LORD. But Abel brought fat portions from some of the firstborn of his flock. The LORD looked with favor on Abel and his offering, but on Cain and his offering he did not look with favor. So Cain was very angry, and his face was downcast. (Genesis 4:2b-5)

Look at the difference between the two: Abel easily gave exactly what God wanted because he didn't worship it, but Cain brought what he (Cain) wanted to bring and kept back what he loved. Many of us have what I call the *Cain Syndrome;* that is, we give to God what *we* want to give—not what He asks for! We get angry at God for asking us to sacrifice the thing we love. Moreover, just as Cain did, we get angry at God for not being happy with what we decided to give Him. For example, many people say, "Well, I gave God my breakfast this morning." But actually, they did not want breakfast anyway. However, when the afternoon snack comes by, they are not about to give that up, even if they are not hungry! They look through the Weigh Down Workshop[†] book for some ideas about the sacrifice they *want* to give. Yes, they will cut their food in half—they will probably end up eating both halves, but they *will* cut the food in half—and they are angry at God because they have not lost weight!

My guess is that if you exhibit the Cain Syndrome, you will also act in the same way toward your co-worker, boss, pastor, or client as you do toward God. You will give these people only what you want to give or what you have decided they need, even if that is not exactly what they want.

The Cain Syndrome is evident in many marriages, too. Married people may do the same with their spouses under the guise of sacrificing. For example, a husband may agree to please his wife with a date but then considers his own preferences—not those of his wife—in making plans for the evening.

A wife may cook a wonderful meal, supposedly to please her husband, but be unwilling to submit to his sexual wants. Just like Cain, she is angry at the husband's seemingly ungrateful attitude for the sacrifice she decided to make for him.

Look at it this way. If an army officer complied with eight out of ten orders, would you say he was obedient? After all, eighty percent of his senior officer's requirements were met. The answer is no. The eight orders completed were just those that came naturally anyway. Not obeying two out of the ten commands reveals a rebellious, disobedient spirit in that officer (sacrifices of convenience).

Obedience is tested only when we confront something we don't want to do. 1 Samuel 15:7–23 tells of God ordering King Saul to totally annihilate an enemy. Through Samuel, God told Saul,

"Now go, attack the Amalekites and totally destroy everything that belongs to them. Do not spare them; put to death men and women, children and infants, cattle and sheep, camels and donkeys." (1 Samuel 15:3)

Saul did go to battle. He did *most* of what God had commanded, yet he spared Agag, the king, and took home some cattle and sheep. Did Saul obey or disobey God? Look at the text.

Then the word of the LORD came to Samuel: "I am grieved that I have made Saul king, because he has turned away from me and has not carried out my instructions." (1 Samuel 15:10–11a)

Samuel confronted Saul, asking, "Why did you not obey the LORD?" and Saul tried to pass his actions off as obedience. "But I did obey the LORD," Saul said. "I went on the mission the LORD assigned me" (1 Samuel 15:19,20a).

Saul, you see, had the Cain Syndrome. He did the part of the command that came naturally—going to war—but where Saul's will differed from God's command, Saul chose his own way. God did not credit Saul with obedience, even though he had been victorious in battle and had carried out a large percentage of the commandment.

In the same way, God did not acknowledge Cain's offering. God knows our hearts. Even though we give God some of the food—the convenient food we want to give Him—that is not being obedient to Him. *He is asking you to go to the next level.* Do not hold out. Rather, give Him everything He wants. With this as your heart's goal, you will not want to "kill" the Abels of this world. You will want to find them and imitate their behavior. You will show honor to those who have given their firstfruits to God and have obtained favor. You can get this acceptance, too! We do not have to get angry at someone else, hate someone else, mock someone else, or murder someone else. Instead of sabotaging a co-worker or trying to find a way of making a passionate person of God's feel stupid, we, ourselves, can give our heart, mind, soul, and strength over to God. Then we, too, will find this same acceptance.

The stronghold of control

It is sometimes difficult to tell that controllers are not on the right bandwagon. They look the most righteous of all the sinners. After all, they devote their heart and soul to working on cleaning up the "world." They object to bad music, and they refuse to patronize businesses that support immoral activities. They try to get their spouses to do "righteous" activities and really rant and rave if they do not get to go to church. They monitor all the foods in the house and the lunch sacks. They *must* be righteous! Homemade bread, water filters, and anything "not clean" is the next topic to study. The children are trained well.

They also monitor parties and holidays. And they usually find themselves pulling back from the world, and adopting a Puritanical lifestyle. After cleaning up the environment at home, then there is endless energy to clean up the school, the church, and the government.

Now, any one of these activities may be fine—but it is the heart we should examine. The person devoted to cleaning up what is *outside* their own heart is *not* doing what Christ did. Christ loved and obeyed the Father and taught others to do the same. One way turns people away from desiring Christianity and spawns rebellion in the spouse and children. The right way—staying focused on loving God with all your heart and your neighbor as yourself—will make you a magnet and will convert many.

"The wise woman builds her house, but with her hands the foolish one tears hers down." (Proverbs 14:1)

You can encourage change quietly. God himself has remained invisible. Why can't we back up a little and trust God to change others' hearts? "Make it your ambition to lead a quiet life . . . to work with your hands . . . so that your daily life will win the respect of outsiders . . ." (1 Thessalonians 4:11,12). "Wives, in the same way be submissive to your husbands so that, if any of them do not believe the word, they may be won over without words by the behavior of their wives, when they see the purity and reverence of your lives. Your beauty should not come from outward adornment, such as braided hair and the wearing of gold jewelry and fine clothes. Instead, it should be that of your inner self, the fadeless beauty of a gentle and quiet spirit, which is of great worth in God's sight. For this is the way the holy women of the past who put their hope in God used to make themselves beautiful. They were submissive to their own husbands, like Sarah, who obeyed Abraham and called him her master. You are her daughters if you do what is right and do not give way to fear" (1 Peter 3:1–6).

Let go of fixing anything outside yourself. Take all that energy, and focus on scrubbing down your own heart. Then, teach the next person the same principle. If you are sure you have pulled the plank out of your eye, then perhaps in love you can pull the speck out of someone else's eye.

Dead-end path—Passion seekers

This road draws weary travelers who are either looking for passion or trying to numb the path of guilt using sex, homosexuality,

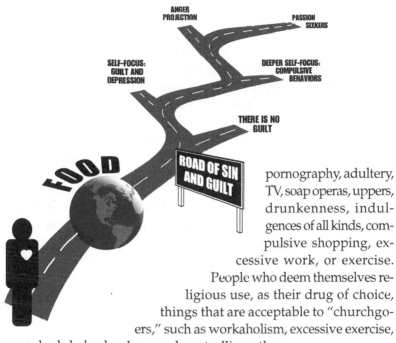

pornography, adultery, TV, soap operas, uppers, drunkenness, indulgences of all kinds, compulsive shopping, excessive work, or exercise. People who deem themselves religious use, as their drug of choice, things that are acceptable to "churchgoers," such as workaholism, excessive exercise, over-scheduled calendars, and controlling others.

Once again, there is nothing wrong with looking for passion. The problem is where we direct the passion. There are many things listed here, but our stand should be made clear. God provides for sexual pleasure just as He provides for food pleasure, but He also sets boundaries. Wanting more than what is in these parameters reveals lust and greed. It also reveals the lack of trust in God to provide for our needs and wants. If these desires are not directed the right way, we will exhibit some behaviors that demonstrate a lack of contentment in our heart. Imagine our hands grabbing for more, rather than calmly waiting—palms up—for our share to be provided by God. Job was a righteous man. He loved and trusted God so much. In Job 31:1, he said: "I made a covenant with my eyes not to look lustfully at a girl." There are several lists of evil desires in the Bible. Here is one:

The acts of the sinful nature are obvious: sexual immorality, impurity and debauchery; idolatry and witchcraft; hatred, discord, jealousy, fits of rage, selfish ambition, dissensions, factions and envy; drunkenness, orgies, and the like. (Galatians 5:19–21a) We cannot leave these desires in our hearts. There is no room for both. God cannot dwell with unclean desires. They are like oil and water—they do not mix. You cannot put new wine in old wineskins, or they will burst. The house needs to be cleaned out before God can dwell there. In other words, God is love, and love will not mix with the hate left in your heart.

Ephesians 4 refers to the continual cycle of indulgence which becomes stronger and stronger. The person can become hardened to the point that he does not care. Many times this person will start longing for additional indulgences and find himself compulsively shopping, addicted to soap operas, addicted to money, pornography, sexual sins and lusts, adultery, television, computers, or their job. Some just find themselves more deeply rooted in just one indulgence. Many of these behaviors are deceptive because we think we are not controlled by them, but they lead down a highway to death of our heart for God. It is hard to see ourselves. The Bible is one of the few mirrors left in this world to show us what we really look like in the heart.

The most deceptive path is the frequently-travelled "Busy-Busy" road. It can almost appear righteous. We use our own strength to get as busy as we can so that we numb ourselves. If we ever stop long enough, we feel the pain. So we just fix that by getting busier— our drug of choice. If God ever stops us and makes us bedridden so that we cannot stay busy, then the pain surfaces and our consciences hurt.

Others may find themselves addicted to gossip. It feels so good to tear others down in order to make ourselves feel better. Gossipers are prone to feel more self-righteous than their friends who chose other wrong paths, such as taking drugs, to cope with their guilt.

The parable of the four soils warns us: "The seed that fell among thorns stands for those who hear, but as they go on their way they are choked by life's worries, riches and pleasures, and they do not mature" (Luke 8:14).

We do not want life's worries, riches, and pleasures to come in and rob us of this acceptance by God and keep us immature.

The Narrow Path

It all boils down to the fact that we are looking for acceptance—which is a *feeling*. It is a warm, loving feeling high up in our heart. Guilt is an ugly feeling, and we may be trying all the wrong things to get rid of it.

Turning to God brings a rush of joy; where depression was once dominant, in its place is now a heart full of unspeakable happiness. There will always be a one-to-one ratio between joy and obedience to God. Antidepressants are not the prescription I recommend. It has to be a genuine repentance with a pure heart.

The pure heart

One of the problems that rises to the top of our heart from the desert heat is the lack of the pure heart. Could it be that you have pursued a relationship with God without a pure heart? Have we pursued God just to get Him to do what we wanted Him to do?

Did you come to the program on your own terms, determined to do only the things you wanted to do, still expecting God to give you weight loss? Once you had a decent amount of the fat removed, did you lose your focus because a focus on Him was not your goal, but rather a means to an end—weight loss? Without a pure heart, you are the ruler of the relationship—not God! If the relationship is with a dog, you are the master. But if you have a relationship with a god, especially *the* God, then He is the master and you are the slave.

Some people love things and use people; others love people and use things. Some people love God and enjoy His things; some people love God's blessing and use Him. God knows when you do not have a pure heart. Weight loss is a fine thing, but more than that, God wants you to look to Him as your deliverer. His goal is to use your desire to be free of bondage to food as a basis for an enduring relationship with Him. He wants you to give your whole heart to Him—not to turn from your lover (food) for only a few days, but forever. He wants you to undertake a true, *spiritual* fast that means forever doing away with this prostitution of your heart for food. See Isaiah 58 for this dialogue.

Those in this category may have lost weight and then stopped losing before reaching their weight-loss goal. They say that they have lost enough weight to be socially acceptable; therefore, the remaining excess pounds don't bother them much anymore. That attitude is wrong for two reasons.

1. These people came to the Lord for what they wanted, weight loss, and not for what He wanted, pure-hearted obedience out of love for Him.

2. They cared more about the praise of men than the praise of God, so that once they met their heart's goal (the praise, or at least not the reproach, of man), they lost their motivation.

The people with pure hearts will keep losing weight, for they stop focusing on their weight and food, and, instead, delight in pleasing God by being obedient and by focusing only on His approval. Likewise, when they mess up, they immediately repent and start over because, once again, they love God so much that they fear His disapproval (the turning of His face from them) as much as they love His approval. They lose their guilty feelings by being obedient. In fact, they lose themselves in God.

What would have happened if Cain had changed his ways? What would have been his behavior if he had decided to change (repent and turn back with a heart to God)?

He would have recognized that he was at fault—not God and certainly not Abel. He then would have looked closely at Abel's heart and tried to imitate the heart that is purely in love with God. Then he would have asked God to forgive his old heart of selfish love. Finally, he would have proved his change of heart by bringing the right sacrifice the next time. No anger toward God and Abel. No playing god by murdering his brother—literally with a deadly weapon or figuratively with ugly words. No jealousy toward a man who innocently gave his heart and, therefore, his pure sacrifice to God. No getting busier out in the fields just to get rid of the pain of rejection by God, and no believing there was no guilt. There would be no substance abuse or numbing agents. There would be no pursuit of counterfeit acceptance—through sympathy or men's approval.

There would be no worldly sorrow—sorry that you just got "caught"—but godly sorrow that brings a 180-degree change so that your mind and heart return to the Father and leave the love of food.

No, the result would have been true repentance that brings acceptance by the best looking, most talented, richest, most powerful being in the universe, the Great I Am. Now, *that* is how you build solid self-esteem! You can master this choice of truly repenting and giving your heart over to the Father. You must master it, because you were made to go down this narrow path and through the narrow door, which gets easier with every pound lost, because now, you see, these are actually pounds of disobedience!

> "Enter through the narrow gate. For wide is the gate and broad is the road that leads to destruction, and many enter through it. But small is the gate and narrow the road that leads to life, and only a few find it." (Matthew 7:13,14)

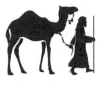

THE TEMPTATION

Are you still having to fight temptation to overeat? The temptation is not based on a physiological feeling or craving. Rather, it is that *desire eating* feeling again. If you are still struggling, please go back and read the "Help! I Feel Hungry All the Time" chapter. This will help. Remember, you are hungry for something much deeper than food. Food will never satisfy this craving for joy and comfort and meaning to the soul. The reason salts and sweets are the typical choice for the binge is that the body is full, therefore, the taste buds on the tongue are dulled. Salts and sweets are about the only foods you can sense. As you approach a 2,000 to 10,000 calorie binge, you literally cannot taste anything. You can hardly even taste the most highly flavorful bacon in a binge. Food will not satisfy. You must try going to God.

I can remember the last time I had a real temptation to binge. I call this the ballet story. I was tired and alone on the weekend. This is the perfect setup for Satan and for true testing of the heart. I was tempted to binge, for I was bored and depressed and had a strong empty feeling. I can remember the strength of the pull of this temptation. The undertow of desire for gratification or indulgence has incredible power or pull if we let it.

I did the right thing: I cried out to God and told Him everything. "God, what I really want to do is go into the kitchen and cook a pan of brownies and eat a big mixing bowl of ice cream with hot fudge and pecans and the pan of brownies. And I would like to finish off the salsa and chips while the brownies are cooking. Now, God, in case you haven't eaten these foods in a while, I would like to remind you that the salsa and chips are great. The brownies taste so good raw or baked, and the half-gallon of ice cream (rocky road) is just wonderful. And it makes me happy to do this while everyone is out of the house. So my question is: 'God, can You do better than that? Can You make me feel better than a binge?'"

God, can You do better than that? Can You make me feel better than a binge?

Well, before I got the prayer out of my mouth—have you seen the scripture, "Before they call I will answer; while they are still speaking I will hear" (Isaiah 65:24)? Anyway, before I got the words out of my mouth, the phone rang. I was tired, but I decided to get the phone anyway. It was dead on the other end. I thought that was strange. Then I remembered my prayer and knew that God was providing a way of escape just for me, as He promised in 1 Corinthians 10:13:

No temptation has seized you except what is common to man. And God is faithful; he will not let you be tempted beyond what you can bear. But when you are tempted, he will also provide a way out so that you can stand up under it.

I starting crying because God had provided many creative ways of escape, but He had never called me on the phone before. I was moved. (My good friends at the Weigh Down Workshop[†] reminded me that God might have called me on the phone, but He also hung up on me!) Oh, well! It was not over yet. In my mind came, "Put on a musical tape." I felt that this was God's leading; therefore, I assumed that the only music He listened to was Christian music—but I could not find any Christian tapes in the pile of tapes. My eye caught sight of a tape on the floor, and I just knew that this was the tape. I did not even look at the title. As soon as I put the tape in, the song started at the beginning of a song that mentioned a love that has existed even before creation itself—longer than fishes, birds, or stars. Not only had God inspired this song—I know He was singing of His love to me.

Well, of course I started crying as my heart welled up inside. I did my ballet (which is no ballet), but it was my ballet I had to offer before the Lord. I curtsied before Him and imagined myself dressed in pure white. I imagined Him extending the King's scepter of approval to me.

The song "Longer" by Dan Fogelberg was in the middle of the tape. What are the odds of the song's starting right at the beginning, and what are the odds of this new equipment—that is still too technical for me to run—to be on an endless loop of this one song?

Before I could get the prayer out of my mouth, God was showing how He could provide instant gratification better than the world!

Did God do better than the binge? You tell me. My heart was so full of love. There were no guilt feelings from bingeing again when I knew that I did not need the food. By the way, the guilt feeling is located in the gut—down low—and it feels terrible. I had a very happy feeling. That feeling is up high—near the heart— and it gives energy. I had lots of energy to dance and sing to God and then to clean the kitchen and get the Halloween decorations out.

I just have to tell you to go to God and ask the Creator of feelings whether He can give you better feelings than the world can. What God can provide is as instant as the binge. Before I could get the prayer out of my mouth, God was showing how He could provide instant gratification better than the world!

Oh, if only I could talk you into going to God for all that you want and need—in place of food, alcohol, drugs, tranquilizers, antidepressants, tobacco, TV, pornography, power, gossip, shopping, materialism, the love of money, or the praise of people. When we leave God out of our lives, what we are left with is an endless black hole. Food never gives back—it only takes. God always gives back.

So the best advice for a temptation is: go to God, ask for help, and ask Him to fill you up better than the world (alcohol, antidepressants, food, attention from man, etc.) can. What I found out is that He loves the challenge and He loves to show off! After all, He has so much to give.

> Hear, O my people, and I will warn you—if you would but listen to me, O Israel! You shall have no foreign god among you; you shall not bow down to an alien god. I am the LORD your God, who brought you up out of Egypt. *Open wide your mouth and I will fill it.* (Psalm 81:8–10)

Open wide your mouth and He will fill you, and this *feeling* you are searching for will be perfect. Just like sex within marriage, food within hunger and fullness is perfect. Going to God to get this *feeling* we all search for is *so right!*

After calling out to God, the desire to go to the food was gone. This is the grace that God has so freely offered us—that if we want Him, He "will remove the names of the Baals [false gods] from her lips" (Hosea 2:17a).

> I will betroth you to me forever; I will betroth you in righteousness and justice, in love and compassion. (Hosea 2:19)

God's grace of a covenant relationship is so inviting that He will take the love you had for food out of your heart and give you a new heart of love for Him. Food loses its tempting allure if you look at it this way.

You have heard me say what your responsibility is. "Therefore, O house of Israel, I will judge you, each one according to his ways, declares the Sovereign LORD. Repent! Turn away from all your offenses; then sin will not be your downfall. Rid yourselves of all the offenses you have committed, and get a new heart and a new spirit. Why will you die, O house of Israel? For I take no pleasure in the death of anyone, declares the Sovereign LORD. Repent and live!" (Ezekiel 18:30–32).

But also, if you want this heart of love, this passion and feeling to all be directed toward *Him*, then pray for it! God can *give* you a "new heart." That is right—*give you*—a new heart if you want it. "The LORD your God will circumcise your hearts and the hearts of your descendants, so that you may love him with all your heart and with all your soul, and live" (Deuteronomy 30:6).

He can put life into dead men's bones . . .
He asked me, "Son of man, can these bones live?" I said, "O
Sovereign LORD, you alone know." Then he said to me, "Prophesy to these bones and say to them, 'Dry bones, hear the word of
the LORD! This is what the Sovereign LORD says to these bones: I
will make breath enter you, and you will come to life. I will at-
tach tendons to you and make flesh come upon you and cover
you with skin; I will put breath in you, and you will come to life.
Then you will know that I am the LORD.' "
So I prophesied as I was commanded. And as I was prophesy-
ing, there was a noise, a rattling sound, and the bones came together, bone to bone. I looked, and tendons and flesh appeared
on them and skin covered them, but there was no breath in them.
Then he said to me, "Prophesy to the breath; prophesy, son of
man, and say to it, 'This is what the Sovereign LORD says: Come
from the four winds, O breath, and breathe into these slain, that
they may live.' " So I prophesied as he commanded me, and
breath entered them; they came to life and stood up on their feet
—a vast army.
Then he said to me: "Son of man, these bones are the whole house
of Israel. They say, 'Our bones are dried up and our hope is gone;
we are cut off.' Therefore prophesy and say to them: 'This is what
the Sovereign LORD says: O my people, I am going to open your
graves and bring you up from them; I will bring you back to the
land of Israel. Then you, my people, will know that I am the
LORD, when I open your graves and bring you up from them. I
will put my Spirit in you and you will live, and I will settle you
in your own land. Then you will know that I the LORD have spoken, and I have done it, declares the LORD.' " (Ezekiel 37:3–14)
Then we will all know in the end that grace is so big that God has
done it all! God can not only put life into our bones—He can do
better than a binge!

Dealing with Temptations

Situations	Responses
1. It comes when you least expect it...	so learn to expect it and pray the Lord's prayer daily. (Lead me not into temptation, but deliver me from the evil one.)
2. It comes when you are vulnerable...	so try to keep rested. Flee the scene. Know your temptation times and locations. Know the "lies" that get you.
3. It comes when you have lost your purposeful focus (on God and His will) and have replaced it with depression and self-pity...	so keep your mind off of yourself and getting your own needs met; rather, keep it on praising God for meeting your needs.

If you have wandered from the hour-to-hour, day-to-day seeking for and receiving acceptance from the Father, you will be left vulnerable and strongly tempted. (The neediness you feel is normal if you have wandered.)

Wake up, and be ready for the fork in the road.
You have two choices—one leads to life, and one leads to death.

Run to Food

Running to the world will only lead you away from giving your heart to God.

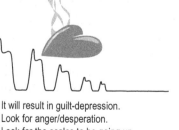

It will result in guilt-depression.
Look for anger/desperation.
Look for the scales to be going up.
The food will never fill up this need.
You will remain needy, because food
  cannot love you back.

Run to God

Cry out to God. Look for your way of escape. He will fill you up, and the desire eating will leave. A word from the Bible (God) may make your heart pound.

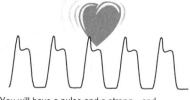

You will have a pulse and a strong—and
  growing stronger—heartbeat for the Lord.
Look for your jewels.
Look for the scales to go down.
Acceptance floods in, and the temptation is
  over for now.

PHOTOCOPY AND CARRY THIS WITH YOU AS A REMINDER

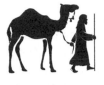

WAYS OF ESCAPE

God knows things that only you and He would know about—private, secret, extremely special, personal things. The desert is a tremendous place of learning, growing, and seeing God's grace and mercy. Some of the most exciting testimonies of His presence and His love for us come in the forms of *ways of escape* and jewels.

A way of escape is based on the verse in 1 Corinthians 10:13 that says, "No temptation has seized you except what is common to man. And God is faithful; he will not let you be tempted beyond what you can bear. But when you are tempted, he will also provide a way out so that you can stand up under it." We take this verse literally; we believe that God will provide a way out from a temptation. Therefore, when I know I am not hungry and just want to eat anyway, then one of the ingeniously creative things God does is to provide me with an escape route. My job is to be alert and take advantage of it! At first, you may not even recognize that God just helped you until after the fact. But you will become more skilled and more observant as time goes on.

Some of the ways of escape that Weigh Down Workshop[†] participants share are downright funny. But I believe that God has a great sense of humor, and He enjoys these creative quests as much as you do. One lady wrote a letter to tell us about an adventure she had one day. She was not hungry but decided to eat a Twinkie anyway. Just as she was about to eat it, an alarm went off. An ambulance came, then a fire truck, then a policeman, and they evacuated her home. She stood outside while they determined that it was a false carbon monoxide poison alarm. After the authorities let everyone go back inside, she discovered that the cat had eaten the Twinkie! Isn't that great? God will go to great lengths to help us on this journey, and it is humbling to realize that He cares so much to provide us with these second, and sometimes third, chances to obey. Unfortunately, we can be stubborn and determined to eat anyway. Then He just shakes His head.

There are many more—cigarettes that get wet, the store running out of the item that you were about to purchase that you really did not need, or the car running out of gas or breaking down on your way to do something that you should not.

The list goes on and on, but here is another cute example of someone in a food temptation. I knew a lady who shared with me a story about a family reunion. She said she was well known for her homemade peach ice cream—so well known, in fact, that she was afraid she wouldn't get any. She knew how quickly it would disappear, so she thought she would sneak over and get the first bowl. Keep in mind that she was not hungry, just afraid she would miss getting a bowl. She did not go unnoticed, and before she could get her bowl dished up, a line had formed behind her. She ended up serving twenty-eight bowls of ice cream! She laughed as she told the story, but she also praised God for His creativity in helping her out.

The ways of escape almost seem to fall into categories. There are escapes that allow you to be distracted from the food, like children needing you, phone calls that interrupt, or guests that drop in unexpectedly. Let me give you a couple of examples of the "distracted" category. One lady had prepared a bowl of soup and had just put her dog outside. Just as she ate the first bite, the dog began barking and got into a fight with another dog (which had never happened before!). As soon as she got back inside from retrieving the dog, she realized that it was her way of escape. She wrapped up the soup and put it in the refrigerator. Here's another one that falls into this category. A mom shared that she had made a Coke float when she was not hungry. But before she could eat it, the phone rang. Then her daughter called her from the bathtub and needed help. By the time she got back to the Coke float, it was just brown, scummy liquid. So she poured it down the drain.

That example of the ruined Coke float leads us into a second category of literally having something wrong with the food as your way of escape—the "disgusting" category. For example, a businessman shared with us about one of the times he was traveling out of town. He said that was always a time of temptation because his company paid for the food, and he was lonely. Eating out gave him a chance to get out of the hotel room and be around people, even if he didn't know them. On this particular night, he was looking for an end to his boredom and decided to go out to a restaurant. He was not hungry, just bored. He ordered a steak, baked potato, and salad. When he got his food, the steak was too rare, the potato was undercooked, and the salad was warm. Rather than getting frustrated with the restaurant staff, he said he just smiled and left them a big tip. We have had so many reports of food being too hot, too cold, the order being wrong, the milk shake machine being broken, or maybe the food just was not available. Here's a great example of that. A lady shared that she was on her way to an annual church retreat.

People have rebelliously gone for more ice cream, saying, "I don't care if it's desire eating I feel. I'm going to get a second scoop anyway."

She knew the area of the retreat well since she had been there several times. In fact, she knew the area well enough to know where the best blackberry cobbler she had ever eaten could be found. On her way into the retreat area, she stopped at the café that made the cobbler and bought an entire pan of cobbler, not just one helping. She arrived at the retreat site, took the cobbler to her room and joined the others downstairs for dinner. After dinner, she went to her room knowing that she was too full to eat, but determined that she was going to eat that cobbler. When she got upstairs, there was a raccoon in the room eating the cobbler!

People have rebelliously gone for more ice cream, saying, "I don't care if it's desire eating I feel. I'm going to get a second scoop anyway." The next thing they know, the second scoop, for the first time ever, has fallen to the floor.

Here is another example of the food just not being available—the "dislocated" category. A man decided to make a homemade pizza. Without first checking the availability of ingredients, he prepared the crust. When he went to get the pizza sauce, there was none in the pantry. So he decided to compromise. He made up a sauce with tomato paste and spices. When he went to get the meat toppings, there were none in the refrigerator. Being determined as he was, he decided that he could just eat a cheese pizza. Unfortunately, he had run out of cheese! Needless to say, he gave up and threw away the crust. Sometimes God gives us more than one chance to catch on.

I know that some will think that these stories are mere coincidence, but I am convinced that God does care about our littlest victories over food. He is revealing His love for us in these little events, and soon we will see Him everywhere and in everything.

He is revealing His love for us in these little events, and soon we will see Him everywhere and in everything.

Another category of escape is the fact that we sometimes can't get to the food— the "disabled" category. I can remember spending an inordinate amount of time trying to get a jar of fudge ice cream topping open once. It had never been that hard to open a jar before. Suddenly it occurred to me that this was my way of escape and that I could wait a little longer to eat. I have had people share funny stories of their being unable to get a package open. They have even shared how they were so determined to get it open that, when it finally did come open— the food went flying everywhere. That very thing happened to one lady with a bag of M&Ms. She was driving her car and the M&Ms popped right out and went flying all over the car. Obviously, she could not pick them up until she got to her destination. By then, she did not really want eat them, since they had been on the floorboard of the car! This incident fit both the "disabled" and "disgusting" categories, but it kept the lady out of the "disobedient" category. God knows we normally do not care to eat food off the floor. I have heard of popcorn bags and potato chip bags ripping apart and spilling their contents onto the floor. I have even had people tell me that the restaurant where they were planning to eat would close just as they walked in. One lady shared with me that she went to a frozen yogurt place, walked in, found no one working behind the counter, no one in the back, and no customers. She said that her initial thought was that a robbery or some other bad thing had happened. She decided the frozen yogurt could wait, and she walked away praising God for delivering her from the temptation.

God is so good to us and so attentive to our specific needs. He ingeniously uses things that get our attention and help us find Him and see His involvement in our lives. This relationship strengthens as we begin to trust Him more and more. Let me give you another example that a Weigh Down Workshop[†] participant shared when she realized that she was relying on exercise to make her thin. She realized that, in her heart, she did not want to eat less food, and she did not want to turn her heart from food to God. She was overeating, but, to make up for that, she would run on a treadmill every day. Again, there is nothing wrong with running on the treadmill, but she was using it in an attempt to stay thin while being disobedient. She said she was coming under conviction to let go of the exercise and just trust God, but she was afraid. One day she came home from work and heard a strange noise coming from the basement. As she descended the stairs, she realized that it was the treadmill, running all by itself, full-speed, burning up the motor. Lightning had hit her house, and the resulting current had surged directly into the treadmill, causing it to turn on.

As you can see, the desert does not have to be a place of constant misery. It can be an adventure. Everyday I wake up and think, "Oh, God, what neat thing are you going to show me today?" A journey with God will be a trip you will remember for the rest of your life. Do you want to know what is even more incredible? You do not

have to wait until the end of the journey to feel God's love and rewards. He is just waiting for the chance to indulge and bless you. If
you will obey, then He will acknowledge that. How? With jewels or
happies! Every time you pass a test, you will get a jewel. Some are
subtle; it could be just the peace of being in His will. Some are ex-
travagant, like large sums of money from an unexpected source or
an unexpected and long-awaited pregnancy. Jewels that Weigh Down
Workshop[†] participants share range from having more energy, wearing smaller clothes, and eating regular foods, to experiencing freedom and a real spiritual awakening. In the Weigh Down Workshop[†]
program, we actually have a class dedicated to *jewels.* Everyone
brings in a token item that represents a jewel that God has given to
them since the class began. Some of the items are giant pants that do
not fit any more, old diet exchange lists they do not need any more,
bottles of antacids they do not take any more, or a half of a candy
bar they did not want anymore because they were full from the other
half. One lady brought in a washcloth because her weight loss en-
abled her to reach her back. Another brought in a pair of panty hose
because she could actually get them on without having to stop and
rest. One couple brought in a pair of ear plugs; the wife had worn
them at night because the husband snored. But the snoring stopped
when the weight dropped. One teenage boy brought in a photo-
graph of himself on a roller-coaster ride. On a previous visit to that
park, he was too big to fit into the cart!

It says in Matthew 7:9–11, "Which of you, if his son asks for bread,
will give him a stone? Or if he asks for a fish, will give him a snake?
If you, then, though you are evil, know how to give good gifts to
your children, how much more will your Father in heaven give good
gifts to those who ask him!" God knows the best gifts, your favorite
things, and how to indulge you with them. If you will just be patient
and obedient, the jewels will blow you away! Do not be afraid that
if you wait on God, the results will disappoint your expectations. In
fact, He will surprise you beyond your wildest dreams! Begin today
to look for your own personal designed-by-God ways of escape and
rewards for obedience.

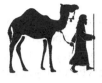

OUTSIDE FORCE VERSUS
INSIDE FORCE

A n outside force is anything that is outside of us influencing what we are doing. It is natural that all of us depend on such a force at one time or another. This outside force can come from various sources to influence our behavior. What influences us after we become adults can vary. When we are younger, the influence starts in the home. It is the thought of the father looking at the report card that influences the time given to homework. It is the mother's Saturday morning room inspection that helps keep the dirty laundry in the basket. It is the schoolteacher's presence that keeps the children from cheating. Later on, it is that highway patrol car sitting alongside the road that makes our foot pull back from the accelerator. It is the possibility of a tax audit that makes us tell the truth to the IRS. It is the force of what others might think or the force of a supervisor walking into our department that makes us arrive at work on time or perform our tasks in a timely fashion. It is the fear of disappointment from the trained technician who weighs us in or the local weight-loss club that threatens to put a picture of a pig around our neck if we have gained weight that makes us stay on our diet. It is a number on the bathroom scales that guides our food intake for the day. It is the exercise guru who tells us to run just one more mile or to do ten more abdominal roll-ups. It is our spouse who might catch us in the pantry at 10 P.M. This outside force makes our heart start pounding when we get caught.

This outside force is the law of good and evil that God set up at the beginning of time. It can either be inside you or it will be outside you. You cannot get away from these ethical and moral laws set up by God any more than you can get away from the law of gravity. God started us off on this earth by giving us an opportunity to choose the law of justice, mercy, and love in our hearts, along with the ability to initiate it ourselves. We missed the opportunity in the Garden of Eden. In the atmosphere of the garden, Adam and Eve did not have an outside force making them behave. What God found one evening when He was walking in the garden, unfortunately, was that the hearts of the free-will agents He had created were missing the inside initiative to be pure in heart.

As time went by, God found a man who did have a pure trust and love for Him. His name was Abraham. Read Genesis chapters 12-25. This man was crazy about God and had such a strong faith that he knew God could do anything He wanted to. God was delighted to find a man who had a heart for Him and trust in Him. However, I did not say Abraham was perfect in *how* he showed his love for God. He tried to "make" the will of God happen by sleeping with his wife's handmaiden. The way people in love with God behave may not always fit our ideas of acceptable behaviors, but God seems to have been patient with Abraham's decision to help get the job done. God knew Abraham's motives. Abraham was even willing to sacrifice his only son if God asked him to. Whatever God wanted was his command. Because of this kind of faith, God considered him righteous. Abraham had the inside force—faith and love. Faith means you think everything God does is cool, and love is comparable to the adoration avid fans show their favorite star.

When God saw Abraham's heart, He sealed their relationship with circumcision, a seal of righteousness. It was like an oath between blood brothers to be faithful to each other for life. It was like marriage vows of devotion between a bride and groom. After God committed Himself to Abraham and Abraham to the Father, God promised to make a whole nation of "Abrahams." In other words, God was so pleased with Abraham's heart of love that He decided to make many Abraham clones, a group of people who had the same heart as Abraham. This spiritual nation was not going to be small in number; in fact, God said there would be as many hearts like Abraham's as there were stars in the sky.

> He took him outside and said, "Look up at the heavens and count the stars —if indeed you can count them." Then he said to him, "So shall your offspring be." (Genesis 15:5)

Diet laws— the outside force

God started fulfilling the promise to Abraham by giving him a child named Isaac. Isaac's son was Jacob, later called Israel. Jacob fathered Joseph, who God sent to Egypt where he became second in power only to Pharaoh. Through circumstances under God's control, the entire family later moved to Egypt, where it grew in number. After they had been there four hundred thirty years, God realized that this large crowd of descendants of Abraham did not have the same heart as Abraham. They had strayed away from the pure heart of their forefathers. God said He would establish a law—an outside force—that would serve until the inside force (Christ in one's heart) was established. If God had not imposed an outside force, they might not have made it until Jesus came. The Apostle Paul wrote, "What, then, was the purpose of the law? It was added because of transgressions until the Seed to whom the promise referred had come" (Galatians 3:19a).

Just before this, Paul had explained:

> The Scripture does not say "and to seeds," meaning many people, but "and to your seed," meaning one person, who is Christ. What I mean is this: The law, introduced 430 years later, does not set aside the covenant previously established by God and thus do away with the promise. (Galatians 3:16b,17)

The hearts of God's people were so rebellious, like wild, bucking stallions, that God had to "corral" them. He put reins on them so, at least, there would be a piece of each heart for Christ to dwell in. The law was added to rein in their transgressions—it was not because

God did not keep His end of the promise. God's law is to His disobedient, hard-hearted, rebellious people what a corral and bridle bits are to a bucking, rebellious stallion. God's law went something like this: "OK, there are seven days in one week . . . devote at least one of the seven days to me—the Sabbath. Now, let's see, I give you all of your money, so set aside ten percent to give back to me—the tithe." So on and so forth.

You see, the people needed a policeman (the law) to get them to show some love, mercy and justice. Jesus' blood brought in the New Covenant. The New Covenant is that the law would be written on our minds and hearts (see Hebrews 8:7–11). Jesus made it possible for us to go into the Most Holy Place so that we could be near God.

Until Jesus came and sacrificed His life so there would be ongoing forgiveness of sins, God could not live in our hearts as the inside force. Holy cannot mix with unholy. Galatians 3:23–25 says, "Before this faith came, we were held prisoners by the law, locked up until faith should be revealed. So the law was put in charge to lead us to Christ that we might be justified by faith. Now that faith has come, we are no longer under the supervision of the law."

That is part of the good news of Jesus Christ—you no longer have to have an outside supervisor telling you everything to eat, drink, and do. You can use your own conscience and hunger and fullness to guide you all the rest of your days! It will become so natural that you will not even have to think about it.

The inside force—Christ

The inside force is the conscience which guides us. This spirit of love on the inside is Christ in us. The law is written on our heart and mind—we do not have to find someone to instruct us or to motivate us from the outside to do what is right, for it is already stamped into our hearts.

Moses describes in this way the righteousness that is by the law: "The man who does these things will live by them." But the righteousness that is by faith says: "Do not say in your heart, 'Who will ascend into heaven?' " (that is, to bring Christ down) "or 'Who will descend into the deep?' " (that is, to bring Christ up from the dead). But what does it say? "The word is near you; it is in your mouth and in your heart," that is, the word of faith we are proclaiming: That if you confess with your mouth, "Jesus is Lord," and believe in your heart that God raised him from the dead, you will be saved. (Romans 10:5–9)

It is inside you—yes, *you*.

Diet rules are the law or the policeman. God has allowed these outside forces from sheets of paper to tell you what to eat. He has allowed fat gram counting and scales to guide you, diet counselors to scold you, family members to shame you, seating aisles to limit you, and clothes to rein you in so that at least you would not eat your way to six hundred pounds! Were it not for the outside diet laws that kept us reined in, there is no telling how big some of us would have become, especially since our hearts were untamed. However, now you are aware of the Good News of Jesus Christ— that His sacrifice made it possible for God to live in your heart to guide you. You *can* cast off the diet laws. You do not have to count another fat gram in your life!

When Michael and Michelle, my son and daughter who are now bigger than I am, were little, I had to have laws (outside rules) to help them dress themselves. My biggest rule or law was that they were to wear no more than four colors on their body at one time. Michelle had more trouble keeping inside these boundaries than Michael, so I would have to send her back to her room to try again. But in other areas of their lives, such as food, I did not have to have outside rules, because I had nurtured the inside force—hunger and fullness—since birth. They could take their Christmas candy to their rooms, and I would find some of it still there at Easter. I did not have to say anything. No outside force—they used their own internal controls.

Speaking of inside guidance, there is no other way to explain the fact that I have been slim for eighteen years without paying for any outside forces to encourage me or pieces of paper to guide me. I have not been on a set of scales to guide me since the early 1980s. I have forgotten where all the calories are and exchanges are in foods, and I am a registered dietitian and have a master's degree in foods and nutrition! I cannot tell you how many fat grams are in peanut butter. I do not exercise formally at all. However, since I am at my ideal body weight, I can run circles around many people. I feel great. I am free of the law. I choose to allow God and His Holy Spirit inside my heart. This God-led heart guides me away from greed and toward using hunger and fullness as internal guidelines. Now, my will and God's will are not in conflict with each other. There are no battles, just internal control.

Help! I have no more willpower

Internal control is not willpower, but, rather, God-power. For most of us, our willpower is long gone. Depending on God's power by praying is completely different. He will make your heart not desire the second half of the candy bar if your stomach is full, and you will be at complete peace from within because you do not want it! Do you hear this? You will *not want* any extra food! The people using their own strength will continue to lust after the second half of the candy bar so badly they can taste it. What is more, they will always have to go against their own wishes—battle after battle after battle.

Self-discipline versus God-submitted discipline

Many people—under the guise of righteous self-discipline—try to run not only their lives but others' lives as well, because they think they can. These people plan their diet and call themselves "successful dieters," but the fruit of this strained life is barren. The family often suffers, because they cannot change the plans of the "self-disciplined." If they have on their plan a low-fat meal, no one can change it, and one had best not get in their way. An example is people with anorexia. These are "self-disciplined" controllers who have not tasted the fruit of "God-control." As time goes on, they will begin to hate their "have-to" exercise regimens and diet rules. They will feel rebellious and will begin to hate the taskmasters named "Fat Grams," "Exercise," and "Food Records." People who keep using their own strength to get by are not new. The prophet Isaiah spoke God's words:
      "You were wearied by all your ways,
         but you would not say, 'It is hopeless.'

You found renewal of your strength,
   and so you did not faint.
I will expose your righteousness and your works,
   and they will not benefit you.
When you cry out for help,
   let your collection of idols save you!" (Isaiah 57:10,12,13a)
People using their own strength eventually become exhausted. The work of their hands does not bear fruit that will last, and they are frustrated because they do not reach *their* goals.

Tapping into inside forces

How do you stop using your own strength and outside forces and begin to be driven by the power of God? You do it with a cry to God for help through Jesus Christ, your Savior. There is no formula for that. I know in my own life that I have been down on my knees many times. I have prayed, "God, get me through this ... I can't do it without You, and I realize I have nothing to offer You in return." I have been on my face on the floor, weeping. I have prayed for God to forgive old things in my life from my youth. I have come before Him, committed to turn from my old ways, and I have obeyed Him. However, not one person is going to look like the next person in doing all these things. Sometimes it would only take moments, and God would hear my prayer and answer me in the form of peace through my tears and power through His Spirit. In times like these, God has led me through dialogue in His Word to reassure me of His love and blessings. I would hear Him whisper, "*Gwen* . . .

   I will make your battlements of rubies,
      your gates of sparkling jewels,
      and all your walls of precious stones.
   All your sons will be taught by the LORD,
      and great will be your children's peace. (Isaiah 54:12,13)
I would cry some more when I would realize it was the exact message I needed that day. The next thing I knew, the house would be echoing with my songs of joy to God.

   It is truly in the heart. As we have said before, you could have two people eating a piece of chocolate cake; one could be sinning

and the other not. It all boils down to their hearts. One is being obedient to hunger and fullness and is at peace. The other one is not
hungry and just ate anyway. There is no way to see their true heart
by their actions in this case. That is why cleaning up the outside of
the person and living in a supposedly sterile community where all
the women look alike and all the men look alike and the environment is squeaky clean—no TV, alcohol, or indulgent junk food—is
not going to make the heart clean. Someone in that environment
may have an evil heart and someone else a pure one. Two people
could be in a bar and one have a pure heart of love for God and the
next one not at all.

Jesus tried to explain this to the Pharisees, a group of people who
were experts at cleaning up the outside, but their inside was "dead
men's bones," Jesus said. Look at this passage, where Jesus is trying
to confront this concept:

"For John came neither eating nor drinking, and they say, 'He
has a demon.' The Son of Man came eating and drinking, and
they say, 'Here is a glutton and a drunkard, a friend of tax collectors and "sinners." ' But wisdom is proved right by her actions."
(Matthew 11:18-19)

You will never please the people who look only at the outside. Thank
the Lord, that is not our goal! But you will please the discerning
people who look to the heart of man. They do not see your looks,
and the only actions they do see are your acts of love to the Heavenly Father. "To the pure, all things are pure, but to those who are
corrupted and do not believe, nothing is pure" (Titus 1:15a).

Unraveling clean and unclean foods

There are so many children of God confused about what is clean
and unclean to the Heavenly Father. They keep their eyes on each
other so much that they lose sight of what the Father thinks. We
need to have eyes only for Him. As we have pointed out, God loves
lasagna and chocolate cheese cake. If we have not studied His personality, we might all be still eating chicken with the skin pulled off
and lettuce with low-calorie dressing! Too many religious seekers
just give a superficial glance at what the Father wants so they can go

spend more time with their idols.

If we have misjudged the food, could we have misjudged in other areas? A casual glance can make you misunderstand the Father's wishes. For example, a superficial glance at the Old Testament might cause you to think that God likes only wealthy people. God gave Abraham, Isaac, Jacob, King David, King Solomon, Job, all the kings, and most of the great men and women great, great riches.

Ephraim boasts,

"I am very rich; I have become wealthy.

With all my wealth they will not find in me

any iniquity or sin." (Hosea 12:8)

To look rich was equivalent with being righteous. To break the stereotype and help people understand that it was not male or female, rich or poor, or slave or free that was the mark of righteousness, Jesus was born in a manger. He had no college education. He chose unschooled men to surround him as disciples. Everything He taught astonished the crowds. They had never heard such insightful teaching, and they heard it from someone who had not been to the schools. His earthly father was just a carpenter. People could see that He had God's favor and seal of approval, and yet, He was a poor man. Look at this teaching from Jesus:

Then Jesus said to his disciples, "I tell you the truth, it is hard for a rich man to enter the kingdom of heaven. Again I tell you, it is easier for a camel to go through the eye of a needle than for a rich man to enter the kingdom of God."

When the disciples heard this, they were greatly astonished and asked, "Who then can be saved?" (Matthew 19:23–25)

Why were they so astonished that being a rich man was not a ticket to heaven? It was because they did not know what God was looking for. They had studied only the externals of approved men and women of God, not their hearts. It is easy for man to imitate the trappings . . . the outside . . . the looks of righteous people.

But notice what the next verse says about the God who looks at men's hearts. In verse 26, Jesus says, "With man, this is impossible, but with God, all things are possible."

Jesus basically spent his life showing the path of salvation or the path to the Father. Since Jesus hit the scene two thousand years ago, we have messed up again. We have studied His hairstyle, His garb, His living environment, and His occupation, but not His *heart*. Some have gone so far as to imitate the trappings by making an issue of living modestly. They outdo one another in rustic lifestyles, and to look even more righteous, grow beards and wear sandals. Parents homeschool their kids and the wives wear no makeup. Some of us believe that if we have Scripture memorized, then we *really* have it! Do not count on it!

> *We need to imitate the inside of His heart, which says ". . .but the world must learn that I love the Father and that I do exactly what my Father has commanded me"*
> *—Jesus*

There is nothing inherently wrong with some of the modern movements to clean up the environment and to separate us from the world, but there is nothing inherently righteous about them, either.

The outside masquerade may fool your friends, but it will not fool God. He looks on the inside. You could be wealthy and be righteous because God made you wealthy. "The wealth of the wise is their crown, but the folly of fools yields folly" (Proverbs 14:24). Again, "Misfortune pursues the sinner, but prosperity is the reward of the righteous" (Proverbs 13:21). God does not look for rich people. He looks for righteous people, and then He blesses them. They are not all wealthy by modern standards. But God has promised to take care of them, and He has promised that the righteous will never beg for bread. God looks at the heart. You could be a righteous person and live in humble settings because God put you there. God wants us to be content where He places us. "Keep your lives free from the love of money and be content with what you have, because God has said, 'Never will I leave you; never will I forsake you' " (Hebrews 13:5).

Again, there could be two women—one working outside the home and one staying in the home. The one outside the home could be righteous and the one at home unrighteous, or vice versa. One could be the Proverbs 31 woman, who "considers a field and buys it; out of her earnings she plants a vineyard. . . .She sees that her trading is profitable." She has another side business: "She makes linen garments and sells them, and supplies the merchants with sashes." This is a business woman who is focused on her family's needs: "She watches over the affairs of her household and does not eat the bread of idleness."

On the other hand, you could have a woman working outside of the home because her children drive her crazy . . . wrong heart. God could have a woman at home taking care of family needs without bringing in an income, or a woman could be in the home but engaging in all types of indulgences, neglecting her family's needs. God wants the heart of the woman to look to Him—not mankind—for instruction. The woman should always look to her husband for guidance from God on any matter, and she should pray, for God speaks through authority. God will know whether the heart of the woman is dedicated to her family or to herself!

God ingeniously made it this way so that we all as individuals, would have to come to Him to make personal decisions. God will show you the motives of your heart.

The answer—imitate the inside of Jesus

Righteousness may do many things and may have different external looks—but its heart never changes; it always looks to God. Jesus was the closest thing to having the Heavenly Father walk on earth. We need to imitate the inside of His heart, which says ". . .but the world must learn that I love the Father and that I do exactly what my Father has commanded me" (John 14:31a). That is what we need to imitate. Jesus just loved the Father!

We have learned that God wants us to lay our lives down for His children, and Jesus was asked to go all the way to a physical death. That is the heart that God is looking for. The Bible is too fun to read as we learn more and more about the attitudes of the heart and what our actions become as our heart changes. For example, as your heart changes from food to God, you will handle food differently than you did before. The way you eat less food will look different from the next person who is learning about Weigh Down†. Some may eat once, and some will eat several small meals. Some will use small plates. Some will use large plates and then use a carryout to store the rest of their food. Some will throw their food away, and some will wrap it up. Some will eat small amounts very fast, and some will eat small amounts over a twenty-minute period. Some will get down on their knees before they eat, and some will praise God quietly in their heart throughout the meal. There will be only one common denominator among these people—they will be God-focused, their hearts desiring to do the will of the Father!

Many people fight over what worship to God should look like externally—the time of day, the place of worship, the length of worship, the type of music, or what should or should not be said. This was a problem in Jesus' time, too. Read how Jesus answered a Samaritan woman:

> "Sir," the woman said, "I can see that you are a prophet. Our fathers worshiped on this mountain, but you Jews claim that the place where we must worship is in Jerusalem."
>
> Jesus declared, "Believe me, woman, a time is coming when you will worship the Father neither on this mountain nor in Jerusalem. You Samaritans worship what you do not know; we worship what we do know, for salvation is from the Jews. Yet a time is coming and has now come when the true worshipers will worship the Father in spirit and truth, for they are the kind of worshipers the Father seeks. God is spirit, and his worshipers must worship in spirit and in truth." (John 4:19–24)

God loves a loving heart and an honest heart. The ways we worship God will look different on the outside, but true worshipers do so in a spirit of love to the Father and in a genuine way. Put another way, all true worshipers have the same heart, and true worshipers are what the Father seeks. Jesus could have established another set of outside laws for worship, but He did not. Therefore, one person could plant himself in the most spiritual-looking church and be as fake as he could be; while someone else could be sitting in what looks like a dead church and be praising God in his heart and life hour by hour. Jesus said, "The kingdom of God does not come with your careful observation, nor will people say, 'Here it is,' or 'There it is,' because the kingdom of God is within you" (Luke 17:20b,21). We had better hurry up and get out of the business of judging externals and spend all of our mind and strength on getting our own genuine love right before the Father!

There is no formula to get your heart right. You need only to desire it. The rest will be easy. God will guide you. It is necessary for you to go the Father *yourself* to work it out. Never in the entire Bible did any prophet, nor Jesus, nor the Apostle Paul present a five-step formula for giving the heart over to God. Many, many showed their attempts to give their heart over with public testimonies, confessions, and baptisms. They gathered at river banks or at other believers' homes, and they worshiped and gave to the Lord at all different times and in many ways.

If you truly worship the Lord, you will do it twenty-four hours a day. I wake up with God on my heart, and my dreams might even be about serving Him. You will not look for a onetime event or a weekly two-hour formula on Sunday morning. Why? Because you will be out from underneath these laws once you have this love in your heart. The law (the outside force) provided a minimum requirement from God to make the Sabbath (seventh day) holy. "Just one in seven," God cried out when He had to add the law. But under the freedom brought by Christ, we can now worship in spirit and truth all seven days. You could worship on an island. There is no formula for Bible reading. You will just crave it. You could love Him, know all about Him, and have His truth plastered all over your heart and be illiterate. You might be known to give more than ten percent of your money, or you might be led to give money in a unique way. The hearts of the worshipers will be the same, but they may be doing different things at different times. A heart of love for the Father and for one another will bring unity of worshipers.

Now, doesn't this make serving Him just delightful?! God's love is there for all mankind. He keeps His end of the covenant; we need to keep our end. Give Him your heart, and He will purify it.

In conclusion, if you ask for it and desire it, God will put His laws into your mind and heart, and you will be guided from the inside conscience. We no longer call upon our own strength nor strength from outside sources. "But if you are led by the Spirit, you are not under law" (Galatians 5:18). It is on your heart, and it is on your tongue. You have Christ in you, and you can call upon the Lord to lead you not into temptation, but to deliver you from evil desires. For the first time in your life, you will feel like an adult as you move away from being told what and what not to do. You will decide what, when, and how much to eat, using only your stomach and heart to guide you.

Since you have asked Christ into your heart, you will have "love, joy, peace, patience, kindness, goodness, faithfulness, gentleness and self-control" guiding you every step of the way. "Against such things there is no law!" (Galatians 5:22,23). "It is for freedom that Christ has set us free. Stand firm, then, and do not let yourselves be burdened again by a yoke of slavery" (Galatians 5:1).

Listen to me, you who pursue righteousness
  and who seek the LORD:
Look to the rock from which you were cut
  and to the quarry from which you were hewn;
look to Abraham, your father,
  and to Sarah, who gave you birth. (Isaiah 51:1,2a)
Look to the rock—Abraham—and imitate his faith and heart for God; you will join a number that is as many as the stars in the sky!

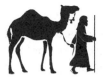

THE PROMISED LAND . . .
DO YOU WANT IT?

G od made a wise decision to start us off with the desert instead of the Garden of Eden. Now the heart was appreciative and non-abusive of the lavish nature of God. No more spoiled children. After forty years in the desert, God was ready for those with the right heart to enter the Promised Land of milk and honey. Those with the right heart can live surrounded by abundance and adore God and not the things around them.

The most exciting part of this whole book is that everyone, whether reading this book or going to the classes, can reach the Promised Land. Since you have learned through the Weigh Down Workshop[†] that there is nothing outside you (spouse, family history, sexual abuse, financial difficulties or anything else) that makes your own heart greedy or angry, then you have control over what you invest your love in. You have the choice to say good-bye to your old love, food, and turn your heart toward heaven. Once you let go of that false god, food, you will never have to walk down the dietetic aisle again. You will never have to eat tuna, drink grapefruit juice, eat cold salads in January, use no-fat salad dressing, eat rice cakes, or drink eight glasses of water per day. As you use your own stomach and loving heart as a guide, you will not restrict yourself to eating only frozen yogurt, grilled chicken or tasteless fat-free cookies. There will be no more guilt or not eating during holidays or at social events. No more rules, reading labels, or buying every magazine with a new diet in it. No more having to eat differently from the rest of the family or shopping for separate foods at the grocery store. No more searching for the perfect diet and no more exchange lists!

The Promised Land is where your will and the will of the Father become married. They are one. You have no desire to eat the other half of the food on your plate. You do not have to worry about where your ideal body weight is. Many people con-

It is going to boil down to one thing: Do you want it?

tinue to lose until they are their lowest weight since high school, if they were not overeaters at that time. Most comments that I hear indicate that the weight reached in the Weigh Down Workshop[†] is even lower than they had expected. If you look at *National Geographic* magazine pictures taken in Third World countries where food is not the addiction—I am not referring to pictures of starving people—you will see that God made people's bodies to be lean. Obviously, women have a higher percentage of fat than men. We must not worry about our bodies.

If you are struggling, it is not for lack of information! You do not need one more revelation or one more sign from God about what to do; you have all the information that you need to lose weight permanently. It is going to boil down to one thing: *Do you want it?*

It is understandable that many people have rejected religion. False religious leaders have turned religion into something that would seem distasteful. Who would want to add long lists of rules to their daily routine? That distortion is what man has established, and that lie is what Satan whispers. We must stop listening to Satan, a creature who never formed a relationship with God because he never obeyed. What does the depraved spirit know? Satan is in the business of making sure God is described as unloving, unmerciful, and unfair. And in the business of telling you that you would make a better "god" if you had half the chance. Do not listen to him.

Listen to this. God is great! Making a practice out of watching what He is up to and how He handles justice, mercy, and love is better than any movie show or bestselling book.

Do I have to be perfect with my eating?

Do you have to be perfect to do Weigh Down Workshop[†]. What if you mess up? Do not worry! Take a fresh look at what God is calling for and take a fresh look at the people who "got it." Let us look at a few of God's favorites and see why He loves them so. When you find this out, you will understand how refreshingly attractive the pursuit of God is and just how possible it is for you to become the apple of His eye, too, and not worry about being perfect.

At a casual glance, you might wonder about these guys who "got it." Abraham—did he not sleep with the servant of his wife? Jacob—did he not cheat, steal and lie to get a birthright? Moses—did he not murder a man?

"When Moses was forty years old, he decided to visit his fellow Israelites. He saw one of them being mistreated by an Egyptian, so he went to his defense and avenged him by killing the Egyptian. Moses thought that his own people would realize that God was using him to rescue them, but they did not. The next day Moses came upon two Israelites who were fighting. He tried to reconcile them by saying, 'Men, you are brothers; why do you want to hurt each other?'

"But the man who was mistreating the other pushed Moses aside and said, 'Who made you ruler and judge over us? Do you want to kill me as you killed the Egyptian yesterday?' "
                                                              (Acts 7:23–28)

Well, if this man of God killed one person, King David killed hundreds. At the end of one of David's war victories, he took off his shirt and danced to the Lord in the streets. Does God condone that kind of behavior?

Rahab, the harlot, lied to the authorities, yet she was among the great people of faith listed in the eleventh chapter of Hebrews. King Solomon amassed a fortune larger than the Vanderbilts', and though He spent seven years on the building of God's temple, he spent fourteen years on his own house. Is that OK with God?

From Abraham to Solomon, none of these favored people of God, whether they lied, cheated, or killed, were questioned for these particular actions or condemned by God. In fact, when David was questioned by the daughter of King Saul as she expressed disgust for his behavior, saying "How the king of Israel has distinguished himself today, disrobing in the sight of the slave girls of his servants as any vulgar fellow would" (2 Samuel 6:20), she was stricken by God so that she would never have children. Not only did God not condemn the people He favored, He protected them by striking their enemies. David's answer explained the relationship he had with God. "David said to Michal, 'It was before the LORD, who chose me rather than your father or anyone from his house when he appointed me ruler over the LORD's people Israel —I will celebrate before the LORD. I will become even more undignified than this, and I will be humiliated in my own eyes. But by these slave girls you spoke of, I will be held in honor' " (2 Samuel 6:21–22).

So what is sin? How could one person kill and it be called murder, while Moses' killing of a man was covered by God? King David wrote about this kind of covering of sin: "Blessed is he whose transgressions are forgiven, whose sins are covered. Blessed is the man whose sin the LORD does not count against him and in whose spirit is no deceit" (Psalm 32:1,2).

The best way to explain this is through the marriage analogy. After you fall in love, the time comes when you and your beloved publicly seal your hearts together with a marriage covenant. These vows are not to be taken lightly; but in reality, there is no way two people know what they are getting into when they say, "For better or for worse" or "Therefore what God has joined together, let man not separate" (Mark 10:9). They just love each other and have passion for one another. As time passes, the wife might forget to do the husband's laundry or the husband might forget to call when he is coming in late from a golf game. Does this wrong offend either person? Of course not! They love each other from the heart, and love covers a multitude of sins. Does it mean that the wife who forgot the laundry loves her husband any less? Why, certainly not.

However, as more time goes by, times may get hard. The couple's environment may become uncomfortable, with the husband losing his job or the wife miscarrying a child. In the rough times, if the wife's heart starts wandering toward her husband's best friend, and her husband picks up on it, and *then* there is no clean laundry the next morning, is the husband likely to be offended? Yes! And he has every right to be. No laundry from the beloved—not a problem. No laundry from the adulterous heart—big problem!

What is the difference? The heart is the difference. One is spiritually healthy, with a great pulse rate, and the other has hardening of the arteries. The hard times reveal the heart, just as the desert reveals ours.

The same is true with our eating. Class discussions often center around this question: "If we take one bite past full, are we sinning?" Our answer is always the same: God does not call us to be perfect—just to not have greed but to trust in Him. Only you would know if that bite represented a heart given to the food or represented innocent extra food. God knows when you are looking through this book to find the easy, natural things to do to get by. He knows when you have positioned yourself so you can "have your cake and eat it, too."

The root problem: Love of food

For I do not want you to be ignorant of the fact, brothers, that our forefathers were all under the cloud and that they all passed through the sea. They were all baptized into Moses in the cloud and in the sea. They all ate the same spiritual food and drank the same spiritual drink; for they drank from the spiritual rock that accompanied them, and that rock was Christ. Nevertheless, God was not pleased with most of them; their bodies were scattered over the desert.

Now these things occurred as examples to keep us from setting our hearts on evil things as they did. Do not be idolaters, as some of them were; as it is written: "The people sat down to eat and drink and got up to indulge in pagan revelry." We should not commit sexual immorality, as some of them did —and in one day twenty-three thousand of them died. We should not test the Lord, as some of them did —and were killed by snakes. And do not grumble, as some of them did —and were killed by the destroying angel.

These things happened to them as examples and were written down as warnings for us, on whom the fulfillment of the ages has come. (1 Corinthians 10:1–11)

Idolatry and adultery is the root sin that God addresses throughout the Word. Likewise, we as humans seem to have a harder time forgiving that sin. God has warned us not to give our hearts to worthless idols, and He has reinforced it with the principle that He has mankind live by: " 'For this reason a man will leave his father and mother and be united to his wife, and the two will become one flesh.'

But God can, and will, overlook our imperfections because of the love in our heart.

So they are no longer two, but one. Therefore what God has joined together, let man not separate" (Mark 10:7–9).

This is all symbolic of the love relationship He has for us. In the beginning, God established a God-mankind relationship. Likewise, among mankind, He created the male–female relationship. These entities are meant to be joined together in love with the attraction that a negative (–) has for a positive (+), like the opposite poles of a magnet. Even though we do not seem to be a likely match with the Almighty God—we live on the wrong side of the tracks, He is rich and we are poor, He is educated and we are not—Jesus makes this union possible by bridging the gap and covering our past wayward heart.

We fall in love with God, and circumcision (to the Jews) or baptism (to New Testament believers) is the public ceremony sealing the love between us and God. It is the outward sign of what is on the inside of us. At first, we do not know what we are getting into. We do not know, at the time we make the commitment, how hard it will be to keep it. However, God is perfect in His commitment. As we grow in this love relationship with God, we will not be perfect. But God can, and will, overlook our imperfections because of the love in our heart. When the hard times hit—and they always do— we must not let our heart wander. It was not made to wander. An adulterous heart is most definitely sin that is not overlooked by God. If your heart wanders, you have broken the covenant with Him. But just as marriage vows do not keep people from getting a divorce, circumcision or baptism does not mean that your heart does not wander. "A man is not a Jew if he is only one outwardly, nor is circumcision merely outward and physical. No, a man is a Jew if he is one inwardly; and circumcision is circumcision of the heart, by the Spirit, not by the written code. Such a man's praise is not from men, but from God" (Romans 2:28,29).

God so adamantly opposes the heart turning away from Him that He gives us many word pictures and biblical examples to teach us never to consider this action. When men and women were caught in adultery in the Old Testament, they were stoned to death. Leviticus 20:10 says that if a man commits adultery with another man's wife, both he and the woman should be put to death. In the books of Ezekiel, Hosea, and Malachi, God said that He "hates divorce." He hates the thought of our breaking up with Him.

God does not want us to forsake our spouse for another, and He certainly does not want adultery to lead to divorce. God hates for anyone to give up on the one to whom a lifelong covenant was made, because it is symbolic of breaking a covenant with Him. But you also saw that adultery was the one big no-no for marriages.

So we need to get out of the pantry. Loving the food (idolatry or adultery against the Lord)—if not repented of—will cause a broken relationship. Do you expect a man to continue a covenant relationship with his wife if she became a prostitute and would not repent? Would your spouse get into bed with you if you were in bed with another lover? I do not think so. God is no different, and it would be insulting to think so. Remember, He describes Himself as a jealous God (see Exodus 20:1–5)!

The key to unlocking the heart

Idolatry is discussed in graphic detail throughout the Old and New Testaments, with Ezekiel 23 being the most explicit passage. In all accounts, Israel entered into adulterous relationships with false gods. In the book of Hosea, God repeatedly called the adulteress back and provided many opportunities for her to return to her covenant relationship with Him. Next He brought punishment on her, and she learned her false gods could not save her. The adulteress returned, but not with genuine sorrow. In all cases, God eagerly waited with open arms for the adulteress to repent and return to His love, but He totally left the outcome up to the adulterous spouse. As I interpret it, we, too, are left with a choice or an opportunity.

Once, when a woman was caught in adultery, her accusers brought her to Jesus to test Him, to see if He would agree to their stoning her. The book of John, chapter eight, tells the story of how Jesus said, "If any one of you is without sin, let him be the first to throw a stone at her." All her accusers walked away, one by one. Jesus told her, "Go now and leave your life of sin" (John 8:7,11b).

In other words, immediately leave your sin and return repentantly to the Father. Indeed, half of the battle is recognizing that, figuratively speaking, you are engaged in adultery. Obviously, one way to find out is to get caught red-handed like the adulterous woman.

True repentance is the necessary next step. John the Baptist preceded Jesus for obvious reasons. We need to clear the heart out to be able to receive the perfectly upright, generous, merciful, spirit of love of Jesus Christ. The book of Luke gives this account of John the Baptist. He went into all the country around the Jordan, preaching a baptism of repentance for the forgiveness of sins. As foretold in the words of Isaiah the prophet, John was:

> "A voice of one calling in the desert,
> 'Prepare the way for the Lord,
> make straight paths for him.
> Every valley shall be filled in,
> every mountain and hill made low.
> The crooked roads shall become straight,
> the rough ways smooth.
> And all mankind will see God's salvation.' "
> (Luke 3:4b–6)

The crowds hearing John asked, "What should we do?" John told them to turn from what they had been doing! Turning not only is the key to unlocking the heart, but it is the key to unlocking God's heart strings.

A wandering heart is devastating to God. The act of betrayal to God is awful. He can overlook imperfection through the blood of

Christ as long as we love Him. However, outright rebellion to His grace and love is different. The act of giving your heart to something else on this earth is in direct violation of the "marriage" covenant between you and God. It symbolizes a love for another, and adultery goes against all that you and God stand for as a couple. This covenant can be renewed upon repentance. That is all God wants from us—our heart out of the refrigerator and back into His presence, with our devotion and love for Him even stronger than before; to place our heart in His hands and leave it there. Permanent weight loss is the result.

Turning not only is the key to unlocking the heart, but it is the key to unlocking God's heart strings.

Love covers a multitude of sins. People have no right to judge God's decision to embrace a repentant sinner. The older brother of the Prodigal Son was jealous that the father had killed the fatted calf for the repentant, returning younger brother, who had squandered all of his inheritance through a very indulgent lifestyle. However, Scripture tells us that there is great rejoicing in heaven when one wandering heart returns home. I bet there are many heavenly parties going on these days!

This much is clear: God cannot transform your heart if you will not give it to Him. But look at people in the Bible who gave their hearts freely to the Father. Their outside may not look clean, but the inside of their hearts sure were . . . They were crazy about God.

Abraham slept with Hagar because He was trying to get the will of the Father done. He was not adulterous in his heart. Later, he raised a knife above his son because the Lord asked him to, not because he was a murderer.

Moses passionately defended the children of God on that early day in Egypt, and he defended God's children and led them to the entrance of the Promised Land. He was not sinning against God.

David so loved the Father that he would dance in the streets even though he was a king. These men were imperfect in men's eyes, but simply being passionate in the eyes of the Father.

When I was a young girl, I wondered about the following statement from God: Just as it is written: "Jacob I loved, but Esau I hated" (Romans 9:13).

Did Jacob not lie and cheat to get the birthright? Is that OK with God? Now, take a fresh look. Jacob was crazy about God, and he would even cheat and lie to get the birthright that made him even closer to God. Esau, on the other hand, was willing to sell his birthright for a bowl of stew! Esau would trade being close to God for food! Does this hit close to home?

"I am the bread of life. He who comes to me will never go hungry, and he who believes in me will never be thirsty."

—Jesus

Zacchaeus climbed a sycamore tree to get close to Jesus (see Luke chapter 19). Jesus' friend, Mary, traded working in the kitchen with Martha to get close to Him. "Martha, Martha," the Lord answered, "you are worried and upset about many things, but only one thing is needed. Mary has chosen what is better, and it will not be taken away from her" (Luke 10:41-42).

These people all had one thing in common: they wanted to get closer to God, and they would do anything to get there. *Do you want that, too?*

The Promised Land is the place to which Moses guided the children of Israel. The disobedient died in the desert and, symbolically, you have allowed God to do such a work in your heart that He has purged all disobedience out of your eating. The Promised Land is a place where you no longer really have to think about eating. You have disciplined yourself to submit to hunger and fullness. Submission is second nature. Your eyes are on the Father. The desert has made you so focused on the Father that if you were asked to march seven times around Jericho, you would just do it. You trust Him, you see that He is in control, and you *love* His control. You can now say that you have risen above the magnetic pull of the refrigerator, and you can stop in the middle of a candy bar with no desire to eat the second half. Going to the Promised Land does not have to take time—it is a choice.

The Word is the "lamp unto our feet" so that we do not stumble. Jesus was the Word who became flesh, and we must continually look to Him for answers about what our God is like and what He wants us to do. That is why Jesus declared, " 'I am the bread of life. He who comes to me will never go hungry, and he who believes in me will never be thirsty' " (John 6:35).

We must behold Christ. If we behold or adore the praise of people, we have missed the mark. If we behold or adore food, we will become a refrigerator. If we behold and adore Christ, we will become like Christ. For better or for worse, *come . . . let us adore Him*. And what God has joined together, let not man separate!

APPENDIX A • TESTIMONIES

Donna Peak—Algood, Tennessee

In eighteen months, I have lost 126 pounds and eighty-five inches. Praise the Lord and the Weigh Down Workshop[†]! I had been overweight for twenty years and had tried every diet known to mankind. God began to reveal to me that my weight problem was spiritual, not physical. One day I received a call from a friend who proceeded to tell me about Weigh Down[†]. I prayed for God's guidance, and He truly worked in my life.

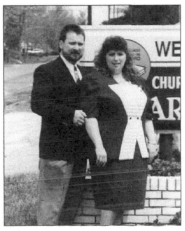

Before

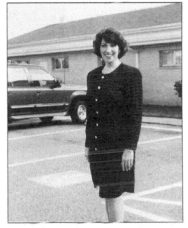

Lost 126 pounds

In the first 12-week session, I lost 44 pounds. However, it wasn't until the middle of the second 12–week session that I came face-to-face with submission and true confession. True confession and repentance poured forth from my heart as I pleaded for the Lord's forgiveness and submitted everything totally to Him. He has truly become my God in every aspect of my life.

My word of encouragement for those of you who have a lot of weight to lose is to not give up. Don't let plateaus on the scales discourage you, because you won't be on a plateau spiritually. As long as you don't give up, there is always hope!

Nathan Kuslansky—Largo, Florida

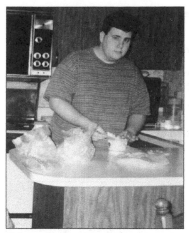

Before

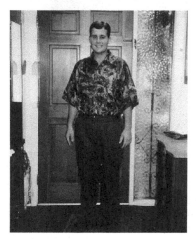

Lost 130 pounds

At eighteen years old, I think I experienced one of the scariest things ever, and that was finding out that I weighed 291 pounds. I was at the doctor's office for the first time in six or seven years when I was told that frightening truth, and I just knew I would never be a thin person. Little did I know that God's timing is the most amazing thing, because the next day a friend's mother was listening to my health concerns and told me that there was a program at church that I could join. I didn't even know the philosophy of the program, but I'd heard how effective it was, so I asked where to sign up.

I soon came to find out that a youth worker I have known for years was an instructor and had been praying for me. After talking to her, I started the program.

Within two weeks, God began to change my life inside and out. The Weigh Down Workshop[†] is literally the best thing I have ever done. My first intentions were to lose weight, but God had much more in store for me than I could ever imagine. I now have the desire to be in God's Word. There is also a constant hunger and thirst in my heart to grow and mature in my Christian walk.

After battling depression and low self–esteem for many years, God began to deliver me from those when I submitted to complete obedience. I have found that when I am willing to die to my will and submit my heart to total obedience to Christ, I am so happy that nothing can bring me down as low as I was.

The transitions taking place in my life made Satan very upset, and he found a way to attack me. Some people don't understand that this is God's way, the only way, and the world has blinded their eyes to the truth. I have found a family in my Weigh Down[†] class that truly supported me and was able to give me the encouragement I needed.

The very best thing I have experienced through the Weigh Down Workshop[†] is the escalation in my spiritual growth. The 130 pounds I lost in eight months are only a side effect and a physical sign of obedience. God has truly blessed me beyond measure, and the only way I know to thank Him is by my obedience and submission. The desires in my heart for growth in Christ can never be fully expressed on paper, but God knows my heart, and I praise His holy name for what he has done for me.

Delores Vaughn—Cookeville, Tennessee

God is so good! I love Him with all my heart. I can't thank Him enough for what He has done for me since May 1994, when I first came to the Weigh Down Workshop.

I had struggled with a weight problem all my life. When I was first really aware of it, I was in the third grade. One day the teacher was weighing everyone in class, and I outweighed everyone . . . even the boys. I was so

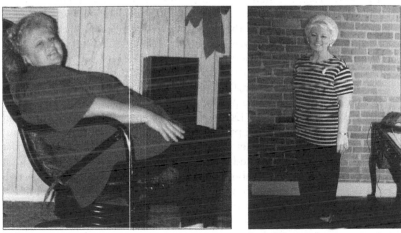

Before   *Lost 160 pounds*

embarrassed because I was larger than anyone. I went home crying and did not ever want to go back to school. I struggled from that day on. Many times I was laughed at and made fun of. Even at a young age, I spent lots of time in tears and praying for God to take the fat away. So I guess even then I knew God was the answer. I had always been a Christian and was raised in a minister's home. I was always taught to trust in God for all my needs, but I didn't know how to search the scriptures for His guidance.

As I reached my teenage years, I tried many diet programs. By then, I really saw the need to lose weight. I had slim girlfriends, and they had boyfriends. I would go on diets and maybe even lose 30 pounds, but I would get depressed and tired of all the liquid drinks and the baked fish, so I would give up and go back to eating. Then I would put the 30 pounds back on, plus more. I did this for years.

When I was twenty-five years old, I met the most wonderful man in the world, and he loved me just the way I was. We eventually married. By this time, I was thinking that I was just the way God made me and I should be happy and enjoy my life. So I accepted a lie from Satan and kept getting larger and larger.

After fourteen years of a wonderful marriage, my husband became ill and, one year later, passed away. At this point I really turned to food without realizing I was going to food for comfort. But God was merciful and was there for me anyway.

About two years went by, and a friend said to me, "You are too young to spend the rest of your life by yourself. It's time to find a nice man to share your life with." I started thinking about what she said. So I began to pray for the Lord to send something positive into my life, since so many negative things had happened. But God had a different plan in mind. He knew I had many areas in my life that needed mending. So He had to get my attention through Weigh Down Workshop, although God knew my physical weight wasn't the only weight I had in my life to deal with. I really believe dealing with the death of my husband and having to face being a single mother of two children, God was preparing me for the Weigh Down Workshop. When I began the program, everything about it fell into place.

I found out about Weigh Down Workshop through a friend who had lost about 70 pounds on the program. There was a beautiful glow about her that was unbelievable. Her joy and excitement about this program just flowed from her! When I called to find a class near me, I was surprised not only to find a class that was about to begin, but I also discovered the Weigh Down Workshop home office was located in the same city where I lived. By this time I was beginning to think maybe God was really in this. I went to orientation and everything I heard that night was music to my ears. I felt in my heart God was finally going to answer my long-awaited prayers. But

I had no idea the wonderful things God had in store for me over the next several months.

God has shown me many things in the time I have been in Weigh Down Workshop. He has made me see things in my life I did not know were there. He has healed my broken heart and is helping me to deal with two teenage children on a day-to-day basis. As an added bonus from being totally obedient to Him, I have lost 160 pounds. I praise God for every ounce I have lost, because it has only been through Him that I have done it.

Many times the desert has been hot, and I have had to lie before the Lord flat on my face in tears, asking Him to help me through. And He was always there. He never once failed me.

It has only been through Weigh Down Workshop's teaching of the scriptures and opening my eyes to God's Word that this change has occurred in my life. I am now more sensitive to the Lord and hearing what He is saying. God has a plan for our lives if we are willing to listen to Him.

I will never go back to my old way of eating. The longer I do as His Word tells me to do—eating when I am hungry and stopping when satisfied—I will never be overweight again. My goal is to be obedient to God and let Him take me to the weight He wants me to be.

We serve an awesome God. He is waiting for us to come to the place where we hunger more for Him to supply our spiritual needs than our physical needs. I praise God for the Weigh Down Workshop's opening my eyes.

My favorite scripture is found in Lamentations 3:22: "Because of the LORD's great love we are not consumed, for His compassion never fails."

DeBorah Stevenson-Payne—Memphis, Tennessee

I came to the Weigh Down Workshop[t] unsure of what was required or expected of me. I knew from our coordinator and the orientation video that it was a weight loss program, but beyond that, I didn't know much more. However, I was sure that if it involved God, I was willing to try. My sister often says that if this didn't work, nothing else could. She's right, and the Scripture bears that out. John 15:5b reads, "Apart from me, you can do nothing." I have lost 38 pounds eating cheeseburgers and "regular" foods, and I've kept it off for one and a half years.

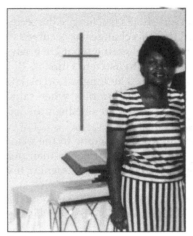

Before   Lost 38 pounds

Kenny Autry—Camden, Tennessee

My sister, Karen, had been trying to get me to try Weigh Down[t] for about a year and a half. I thought, "Why go to this? It's just going to be another diet plan." She just wouldn't quit until I got really angry. Karen was praying one night, telling God she had done everything possible. God told her "No you haven't, go get him!" Karen called me back and promised that if I would go to orientation, I would never hear about Weigh Down[t] again. I said, "Fine, I will go—but I don't want to hear anymore about it."

I went to orientation just to get her off of my back! There was so much love in the class that I signed up.

I am 5 foot 6 inches tall. I weighed 315 pounds when I began the class. I could not sleep at night; my fat would just shut off my air. The only way to get any rest was to sleep in an upright or praying position. It was so bad, I would go to visit someone and just fall asleep. At the time, I was going through a divorce with two small children involved. I was so depressed and angry; it was everyone's fault except mine. I was going to church, but not doing what the Lord wanted me to. Every time I got upset, I would eat; every time something happened, I would eat. For no reason at all, I would eat. I no longer cared if I lived or died.

I have never felt so low in my life—it was terrible!

I had been saved but was not being obedient to God's will. This class helped me to realize how much God loves and cares about each and every one of us. Once I began to study the Word and listen to the tapes, I began to be convicted. The more I studied and prayed, the more God showed me. (The "Emotional Eating" tape got to me; it was like Gwen was inside my head, knowing everything I had been doing and feeling.)

I began to lose weight, but the real change was in my soul. I got to where I could sleep at night, but the difference was the change in my outlook. I realized life is wonderful and worth living, with God's help. My divorce went through, but with God's help I accepted it. My girls eat dinner with me three or four nights a week. The peace and rewards that come with total obedience cannot be explained in words. I am not perfect. I never will be. But a closer walk with God is my life's goal.

My favorite scriptures are in James 1:2-6,13-15, Psalm 34, and Isaiah 40. Both of these last two chapters are very uplifting.

Psalm 40:1-3,11-13 says, " I waited patiently for the LORD; He turned to me and heard my cry. He lifted me out of

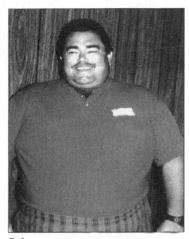

Before

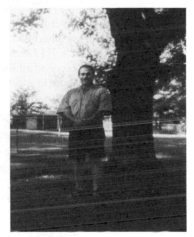

Lost 122 pounds

the slimy pit, out of the mud and mire; he set my feet on a rock and gave me a firm place to stand. He put a new song in my mouth, a hymn of praise to our God. Many will see and fear and put their trust in the LORD . . . . Do not withhold your mercy from me, O LORD; may your love and your truth always protect me. For troubles without number surround me; my sins have overtaken me, and I cannot see. They are more than the hairs of my head, and my heart fails within me. Be pleased, O LORD, to save me; O LORD, come quickly to help me."

2 Timothy 1: 6–11 says, " For this reason I remind you to fan into flame the gift of God, which is in you through the laying on of my hands. For God did not give us a spirit of timidity, but a spirit of power, of love and of self-discipline. So do not be ashamed to testify about our Lord, or ashamed of me his prisoner. But join with me in suffering for the gospel, by the power of God, who has saved us and called us to a holy life —not because of anything we have done but because of his own purpose and grace. This grace was given us in Christ Jesus before the beginning of time, but it has now been revealed through the appearing of our Savior, Christ Jesus, who has destroyed death and has brought life and immortality to light through the gospel. And of this gospel I was appointed a herald and an apostle and a teacher." This scripture has made me realize that if I fear or doubt, it does not come from God. God's Spirit is of power, of love, and of self-discipline.

In thirteen months, God has taken away 122 pounds. Praise Him! Praise Him! The rewards of obedience are endless, as is God's mercy.

Helen Luck—Kalkaska, Michigan

It's the first time in twenty-five years I've worn skirts. I'm a 76-year-old grandmother who weighed 250 pounds. I've dropped five dress sizes so far and lost 64 pounds. If I can lose weight at the age of 76, you beautiful young women who have a full life ahead of you can accomplish the same goal. God's hand is there to guide you.

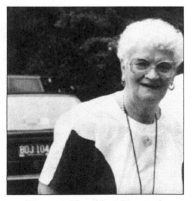

76 years old and lost 64 pounds

Mary Jo Runfola (a former Miss Ohio)—Powell, Ohio

I have been a model and a beauty queen. I was so ashamed of myself as I started gaining weight in my late twenties. I had battled weight since my teenage years. This workshop and the Biblical principles taught by Gwen have revolutionized my thinking about food! I have lost 35 pounds without giving up anything I like to eat. I will never be deprived or starved again!

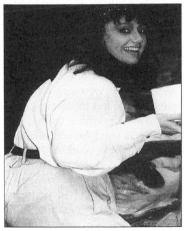

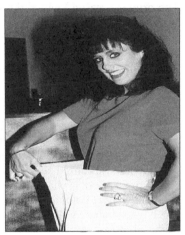

Before   *Lost 35 pounds*

Janice Hoefer—Higginsville, Missouri

I used to drink alcohol quite a bit. I even attended local alcoholic support group meetings because I felt maybe I was becoming an alcoholic. I was having lots of problems with my attitude toward my family, because I constantly yelled at them and was so negative. I took antidepressants and saw a counselor for many months. Your program changed my life. It also prepared me for the hospitalization and near loss of a close relative a month after I began Weigh Down[†]. He was poisoned by overindulgence of alcohol. I gave him to God as we drove behind the ambulance, and I realized how I needed to change *my* life. My relative should have died or had brain damage or something, but he did not. He is strong and healthy, and I know God has plans for his life, just as He does for me.

I had gradually given up my alcohol almost completely when I went to the Weigh Down Workshop[†] convention last summer, but wine was still a temptation. While I listened to the powerful singing at the convention, I felt God's presence all through me, and I just gave it *all* to Him. I have since ordered a glass of wine once when out with friends, and I drank half of the glass and left the rest. That is amazing and a miracle of God working in my life! I am so excited about sharing how my life has changed in so many ways since your program brought me closer to the Lord. I will always be grateful for getting another chance to know God.

Melissa Shepard—Broken Arrow, Oklahoma

The primary reason I joined the Weigh Down Workshop† was not to lose weight. I had an entirely different problem, but the very same root problem as a person in bondage to food. My bondage has been to pull out my hair, literally. You have heard the old saying, "I am so stressed, I could just pull all my hair out!" Well, I really did that. I have had the problem ever since I was eight years old. I am now twenty-one years old. I used hair pulling as a means of escape whenever I was nervous, stressed, fatigued, bored, scared, lonely, or ashamed. My parents took me to doctors, psychologists, and counselors, and I was told it was everything from a bad habit to a form of obsessive-compulsive disorder. I tried several forms of behavior modifications and medicines, but nothing ever worked. I would pull my hair out until I was totally bald on top of my head.

But praise God, He had a different plan! My mother, who had struggled with her weight, got into the Weigh Down Workshop† along with my aunt. She began to share with me some of the truths she had been learning. She said, "Melissa, we share the same root problem and these truths can help you stop pulling your hair just like they are helping me to lose weight." It

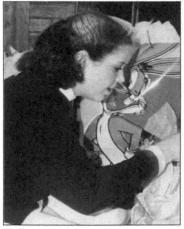

Before

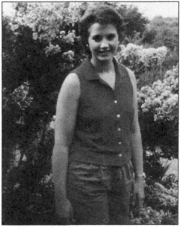

After

all made so much sense. So I started the Weigh Down Workshop[†] in March of 1996. Through Bible study and listening to the tapes, God began to open my eyes to see that I was enslaved by the sin of hair pulling. I realized that I had made it my god and used it to comfort me instead of Almighty God. I repented and gave this stronghold totally to God and He immediately healed me. He took the chains of hair pulling and broke through them. To this day I have not had any desire at all to pull my hair. In fact, the thought of it is repulsive to me. Isn't God amazing!

Gloria and Mary Cameron—St. Thomas, Ontario, Canada

I entered the desert on the coattails of my 17-year-old daughter, Mary. I joined the class in support of her, but I soon realized my own need for deliverance and have lost 15 pounds. God has used Mary's faith and obedience to teach and inspire me. She lost 40 pounds in one year and began wearing a size 5/6.

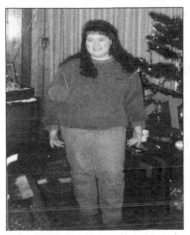
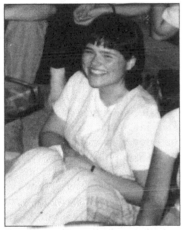

Before   *Lost 40 pounds*

Jill Bass—Memphis, Tennessee

To God be the glory, great things He has done! Seven years ago, I began my first diet and slowly but dramatically fell into an "eating disorder" that controlled my life! For the first two years, I was labeled as anorexic. I had mastered the "art" of starving and exercising. When self-control became impossible (as it always does in *self*-control), I became an "exercise-bulimic," bingeing beyond control, then starving and exercising compulsively to control the weight. I tried vomiting. Praise God that it would not work! I thought about food constantly. I weighed two and three times a day. I concentrated on what I was going to eat and then, after eating it, I focused on how I was going to starve or exercise to make up for it. I could consume more food in one sitting than I ever dreamed I could, then eat nothing for one or two days and exercise for hours. Anything that interfered with this pattern irritated me terribly. My life revolved around this simple cycle.

I am convinced now that I was in bondage to sin and the enemy. Although a Christian, I had closed my eyes to the sin that enveloped me. I was so focused on—and proud of—controlling this weight myself! What willpower I had! How thin I was! How *enslaved* I was! I tried everything—low-fat, no-fat, fiber, eat more, weigh less. What garbage! I even sought secular therapy and Christian therapy when I finally realized that I was on a downward spiral!

Praise God for the parting of the sea! He prepared me for the Weigh Down Workshop† by bringing me to the breaking point! I no longer wanted to be controlled by this disorder. I cried out to Him. He led me to Weigh Down† in an amazing way. I then heard an ad on the radio and called the 800 number to see if there was a session on the *one* night that I could make it. There was, starting the *next* night.

I *knew* then that this was it! I was packing my bags to leave Egypt! But boy, did I underestimate Weigh Down†! This was much more than Biblical truths to help me apply secular principles. This was God's way of eating! What an awesome Creator! Once I recognized the patterns of my behavior for what they were—*sin*—I was on the way to the Promised Land.

After the first session, I knew this was the answer to the bingeing and starving. What I did not know is that God had something in mind that I had never imagined. He wanted to deliver me from another bondage as well—compulsive exercise. I now see that this controlled my life even more than the excessive food or the deprivation of food. I never thought I could give up exercise. That is how I controlled my weight and my *sin*. For seven years, I exercised strenuously for over one hour five to seven times a week. I revolved my days around getting to aerobics. Trips were major stresses because I had to give up my exercise. It has been seven years since I enjoyed a vacation. The longest I had ever gone without exercise was seven days. That was when I *had* to go to Hawaii five years ago. Each day was spent worrying about missing exercise and gaining weight. I recently skipped ten days of exercise without worrying one bit. In fact, God is working dramatically in this area, and I find myself fitting exercise in every now and then. Now I exercise because it helps me to sleep and feel better—*not* because it is *my* method of controlling my weight. My method for that is to obey God's created signals. *He* will control my weight.

At first, I was very fearful of this program. Satan told me that if I obeyed God and didn't do this myself, I would get fat (I did *not* need to lose any weight but Satan had me fearing I would gain weight, especially if I did not exercise). But God's Word tells me that every good gift is from Him; He desires to give good things to His children and reward those who seek Him.

For weeks I craved nothing but sweets when hungry because I had deprived myself for years. Now I let myself eat what I want. I still cannot get enough carrot cake. I often eat a small piece for lunch! For a while, I ate a doughnut for breakfast daily, but now I am back to craving cereal! I am amazed at the small amounts I am eating! It is so much more satisfying to eat one doughnut than a *huge* bowl (double serving) of fat-free oatmeal. Half of a burger and a few fries is *great* compared to a gigantic *plain* baked potato with a plateful of broccoli. I love realizing that God wants me to enjoy eating! He just wants me to eat within His boundaries—which are set up to keep me at the right weight. And that weight is *not* fat! I love not being stuffed, and I love feeling true hunger. I feel like I am discovering these joys for the first time. Most of all, I love the fellowship with the Father that I am experiencing as I grow in obedience and love for Him.

I have lost *some* weight. I am at the weight that I hope to maintain. I believe God allowed me to lose a little to confirm His goodness and grace. He miraculously delivered me from head hunger. He is still working with me on stopping, but He is teaching me mercifully in the desert, so I am completely prepared to live in the Promised Land—free of binges, purges, and compulsive exercise.

My 'jewelry chest' is full of jewels! The biggest is actually having a life that does not revolve around the aerobics schedule. I truly believe that God has even seen to it that other things were happening when I would have gone to aerobics. He often even said to me, "Don't go to aerobics, go home and spend time with me." I did it! That is a jewel! And guess what— I did not gain an ounce by not going!

I love feeling 'normal' in my eating. Going out to lunch and dinner is no longer a battle, but a joy. I even schedule *both* lunch and dinner out in the same day without concern. Before, this was a nightmare because I could consume more than a day's worth of food at one sitting—especially if going out to eat.

Another jewel is having my marriage back. I have only been married for three years. I hit the lowest point of my food/exercise sin during the first year. I have been consumed with food, exercise, etc., for our entire marriage. Praise God for a godly husband who has understood and supported me. I believe that now God has given me an opportunity to be the wife He calls me to be. How often I blamed this wonderful man for my problems, and how often he suffered both personally, socially, and emotionally because of me!

Obedience is another jewel. I am focusing so much more on obeying

God in all areas of my life. In doing this, I have received peace and rest! God is such a personal, unique God, and He has often given me personal 'ways of escape' and nudges to obedience that are just between Him and me. How awesome that He wants to be personal with *me* —an unfaithful sinner. He also wants to take the time to train and correct me. I have grown to value this and not neglect His teaching. I have come to know Him better as Father—in His compassion, mercy, and desire to spend time with me; as Son—in His forgiveness, resurrection, and power over sin; and as the Holy Spirit—in guidance, conviction, and peace! All of these *jewels* are for choosing *His* path!

I praise God for His timing in leading me to the WDW[†]. His timing is perfect. I praise Him now for the years of suffering. Our precious God even turns our sin around for His glory. What a Master over Satan! I can hardly contain this victory. I know there are many women out there with eating disorders and exercise compulsions (*sin*). I hope that I will be able to share God's victory with them. Though the bulimic or anorexic woman has a very different compulsion than the overweight woman, her victory comes from the same place—our mighty resurrected Lord!

Lynda Bessell—Ilford, Essex, United Kingdom

Even though it has not come off very fast—God has been teaching me many things as I lead a WDW[†] group class in England. I have now lost 56 pounds, and I am sure the rest will quickly follow.

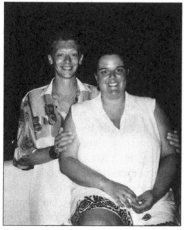

Before

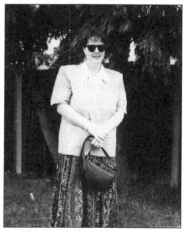

Lost 56 pounds (4 stone)

Debbie Auter—Tallahassee, Florida

I had bulimia for about ten years, ran excessively for fifteen years, counted calories every day (except those days during bingeing and purging) for 23 years, been on every imaginable diet, did the body wrap spa, and joined exercise programs. That is why I don't have a significant weight problem. I have had, however, the worst possible turmoil, degradation, and hatred of self. Since the Weigh Down Workshop^t, I have lost five pounds! Since I stopped purging, I have not gained any weight. I praise the Lord I have been delivered from the obsession with food. I can't begin to express my gratitude to the Lord for giving me this freedom for the last two years!

Sally—Long Beach, California

God laid on my heart that I needed to tell you a little about what Weigh Down is doing and has done for me. Before the program, I had a low opinion of myself and couldn't believe that God knew who I was, let alone *cared* about me! I bought into the lies that I was a horrible person, stupid, incapable, unworthy of anything good in life. Of course, being married to an alcoholic didn't help! I didn't like my job, either. Every day was a pity party. Finally, at night, I'd be alone to pig out on whatever I could find!

At the beginning of the year, I weighed 212 pounds at five feet, five inches. I couldn't go to the beach or hike or go horseback riding. I was miserable! I understood I was giving food too much power in my life. I prayed for release, but I wouldn't totally give up the food to God. The next month, Weigh Down^t began in my church. My life will *never* be the same! I'm working on a new career. I enjoy teaching and helping others improve their lives through a stronger relationship with Christ.

Since Weigh Down^t, my husband has given his life to the Lord, but he still drinks. That, I believe, is next on God's agenda. Our marriage is improving daily as I relinquish my long-standing position as self-appointed head of the household and become the submissive wife. It's really hard, but it's worth it.

So far, I am down to 170 and still dropping, and I've gone from a size 20 to size 14! I would not be the person I am today if I had not let God's Word light up the darkest corners of my heart. Slowly but surely, my life is being restored!

Nanette Newman—Racine, Wisconsin

Thank you, Gwen, for showing me how to love the Father. I know that it is Christ in you that causes me to love the Father when I hear you speak of Him.

After just two weeks in Weigh Down[†], I believed wholeheartedly that you had found "IT." I weighed 310 pounds and lost 40 that first session. When I started a class at my own church, the weight loss ended. But I knew there was no going back. To what would I go back? I had been to psychologists and countless weight loss programs. I knew that those paths were wrong, but, like Paul said, "That which I want to do, I do not do; and that which I do not want to do, I do." (Romans 7:14-15)

As I cried out to God in desperation, He said to me, "I'll give you the victory, but I'm going to take you through some things to show you why you've had to endure this bondage."

I attended Desert Oasis [the Weigh Down Workshop[†] national seminar] and saw God's love with my eyes. I pleaded with God to help me love Him as you do. I can now tell you that I've fallen in love with Him—so much that there is no food that can even rate next to Him!

Before my desert experience, I thought I loved Him. I even believed I'd die for Him. But the verse which says "If you love me, you will obey me" kept haunting me. How could I say that I would die for Him when I couldn't even leave Him a bite of my food? So I stayed in the desert for one year—long enough for God to show me the way He wanted me to love Him—with all my heart, soul, mind, and strength!

Gwen, as I watched you talk about how you loved Him, it was like your hand reached out and grabbed my heart, put your love for Him inside, and put my heart back into my body. I wondered if it was real. After I got home, I was ambushed by temptation. I repeatedly cried and waited. I was scared God wasn't coming! But then He did, and boy did He ever! I put in the last tape of "Freedom for the Captives," and guess what came on when I hit PLAY! It was your special song from God!

His love overpoured my soul! And now, with my heart throbbing, I can say, *"I Love Him!"*

APPENDIX B • CHILDREN

P arents should start being responsive to their infants' hunger at birth. Feed on demand. However, make sure you learn the difference between the cries for comfort and the cries of discomfort of a wet diaper, etc. Mothers who try to finish off a "serving size" determined by a baby food company have just confused the infant's natural hunger mechanism. You cannot see the serving size that is offered by breast-feeding mothers. You have to trust the infant's hunger and fullness mechanism. For this and many other reasons, I suggest breast-feeding for a natural amount of time.

Children who do not have weight problems

It is great for you to let go of control of your child's eating at the dinner table. Your job should be to serve a variety of foods. This way, your child will not overeat. Make sure that they are not drinking the bulk of their calories. Too much sweetened fluid is not good. After counseling for years, I saw that the number one enemy is drinks, especially fruit juices and sweetened drinks—even if the source of sugar is "natural." (I cannot really think of anything sweet-tasting that is not of nature except artificial sweeteners, such as saccharin.) At any rate, the point is that the child will become anemic if their main source of calories is just sugar water, because they will not be hungry for solid food. Provide water or some artificially sweetened beverages between meals. Just one serving of juice could cause a little one to skip breakfast, so save the juice for the meal.

Desserts should not be associated with the meal. In other words, you do not want to set up a reward system of, "If you eat your food, then you can have your dessert." At our house I offered supper to my family. Later that night, if the children were hungry again, I would let them choose what to eat. Sometimes they would choose a dessert, and sometimes they would want cereal. (Actually, most current cereals are really just a dessert anyway.) Or sometimes they would want some more of the supper. Sometimes they were not hungry after supper.

In an effort to try to free you up and help you not to worry if your children do not always eat the "perfect meal," I must let you know that I have tried to stay back and let my children form their natural eating selections. I never monitored amounts. I provided variety, and if I introduced new foods (like some raw vegetables with dip) I would just fix it, set it down on the coffee table in front of the TV and tell them, "Now don't eat this. This is for the adults." It worked every time! As I look back on it, Michelle has never seemed to gravitate toward anything green. That has changed somewhat now—but she is full grown and in good health. Michael has never seemed to like potato dishes. He will eat a few french fries, but they are not his favorite food; and yet creamed potatoes and gravy are some of my favorite foods. Milk and pizza seem to have been the staple foods at our house.

By the way, thin children are as normal as big-boned children. God made them all, and the variety is adorable. Spend your energy on loving one another at meal times.

Overweight children

If your child is overweight when you get this book, do not despair. Try to focus on your own obedience first, and you will make the largest impact on the child in that way. Do not control their eating. Pull back. Teach them the basic hunger and fullness information. Make sure you make them their own personal Weigh Down Workshop[†] box that has their name on it.

When your children say, "But my tummy wants more," and you know it is head hunger, say, "You can have it later." Put the food in a clear plastic bag and put their names on it. Now you know that the children have an empty hole in their heart that needs love and at-

tention. You can provide
this by using an alter-
nate activity. Go on a
walk together or swing on
the ropes together or go play
with the dog or read a book
together. Point out to them later
that they completely forgot about
the food. Show them that they did not
eat that food when they did not need to
eat it, and praise them for this.

Never be a member of the "clean plate club." Try to take focus off
the food for your child and try not to make fun activities center
around making cookies or baked goods. Try doing arts or crafts together in the cold months. Teach him about God and help him develop a relationship with God. Teach him how to pray and help him
at an early age see his prayers being answered. Help him go to God
for comfort when it seems that prayers are not answered. God will
teach your child as you stay focused on pleasing Him.

Appendix C • Body Measurements

I t is important to begin this journey with an open heart and mind. Our major objective is to replace our passion for food with a passion for God, our Heavenly Creator and Caretaker.

Now about those scales!

God is trying to deliver you from bowing down to the "scale god." How sad to think of the millions of people in this country bowing down to this false god to get approval or to see if they have been good or bad! However, if you occasionally want to weigh and record your body measurements, space is provided on the following pages.

Weigh no more than one time per week. As you are learning to rise above the food, learn to rise above the scales, too. Some of you are getting on the scales three times each day! Start using your conscience—your inside force—to tell if you have been obedient or not.

The first two weeks, you can weigh more often so you can see that the program works. After that, however, back off. This piece of metal cannot judge you or make you feel good or bad.

Do not be surprised if your weight goes up if you are disobedient to the stomach.

Do not be surprised if you are a female and your weight goes up when it is time for your monthly cycle.

Do not become depressed if one week your weight does not go down although you did everything right; you are being tested to see if you will be obedient to God even when you do not get immediate rewards.

Do not get depressed if you cannot pull together complete obedience to God in the first few weeks of the program. I have seen every possible combination. Just keep focused on what you are supposed to be doing. Use your conscience; talk to God, and if your weight graph is not going down, eat less food! It is not going to kill you to eat less.

Above all, do not compare your desert walk to someone else's. God has your walk already mapped out; just look to Him for everything!

How fast do you lose weight?

When you eat less food, you will lose weight. The person who eats when hungry and stops when satisfied—not stuffed—will lose weight at one to four-and-a-half pounds per week. This is not four pounds of fat cells—this is fat plus the surrounding fluid that keeps those cells alive. This is the way the body wants to lose weight. We have so much evidence of people who look great because they are responding to the body. People who lose weight rapidly on liquid fasts often have a gray pallor to their skin. Not so in Weigh Down†.

Taking measurements is very important. Every so often, you eat right, yet the scales do not show the drop. You need to just focus on God and look for other rewards from Him. Check your measurements. Sometimes, this delay in the weight loss can go three weeks in a row. But normally, if you have not dropped by the fourth week, you need to be more attuned to your hunger and fullness.

> Woe to those who go down to Egypt for help, who rely on horses, who trust in the multitude of their chariots and in the great strength of their horsemen, but do not look to the Holy One of Israel, or seek help from the LORD. (Isaiah 31:1)

I have seen consistent four-pound-per-week weight losses, and I have seen consistent one-pound-per-week losses. Never fear that you will not get to food, for this God you serve owns all the grocery stores in the world, and He can take five loaves and two fishes and feed five thousand people. So keep focused and keep the faith. Weight loss is inevitable. Before long, there will be *less of you* and more of Him!

Do not get tempted to go back to Egypt

You do not ever want to do anything that allows you to chew more food, whether it be eating tasteless, low-calorie foods or exercising so you can chew more. Determine today to *eat less food*.

Do not let your heart wander to the refrigerator. Read "The Temptation" chapter over and over until it is memorized.

If you plateau for more than three or four weeks, read the "Feasting on the Will of the Father" chapter and make the choice to give Him those last morsels of food. Go to God in prayer.

WEEK

Weight Loss Graph

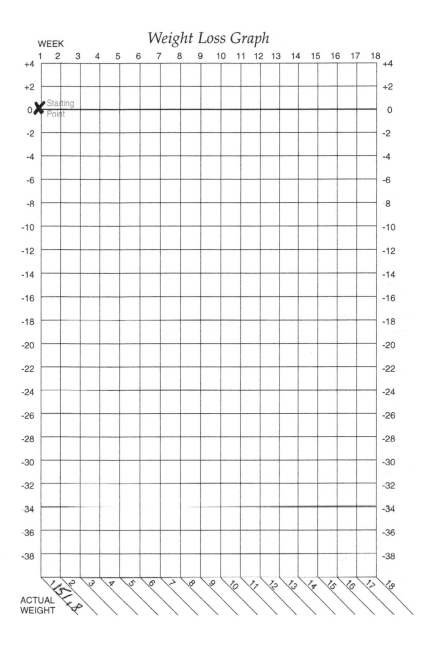

Body Measurement Chart

Date	(Date I left Egypt)						
Chest							
Arm							
Waist							
Abdomen							
Hips							
Thigh							
Calf							
Total Inches							

We encourage you to record your total inches in the spaces provided above. Do not get discouraged if the inches seem to be coming off at a slower rate than you desire. Permanent losses take longer than temporary ones, but they are worth the wait!

Try to measure at the same points each time. For example, measure your thigh seven inches above the kneecap and your abdomen two inches below the waist.

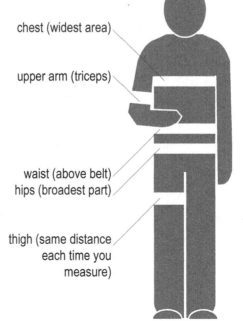

chest (widest area)

upper arm (triceps)

waist (above belt)
hips (broadest part)

thigh (same distance each time you measure)

Appendix D •
Travel Diary

This section is where you record your desert experiences. Use the diary to record insights that God gives you from the Bible. Indicate your victories and struggles. Each week, take time to review what the Lord has shown you from the Word.

1. **Loving thoughts to the Father**—This space could be used for anything. People have shared with us thoughts, poetry, songs, and stories that they recorded in their own Travel Diaries. Pour your heart out in this section if you like to record your heart-felt thoughts.

2. **Heartfelt lessons from the Father**—Use this section to reflect on what God has revealed to you from Scripture. It is our deepest desire that you learn to turn to God as your guide in all areas. Just as you seek Him regarding when and what to eat, you can seek Him regarding when and what to read from His Word. Here are some guidelines to help you with your Bible reading and daily seeking after God:

   • If you haven't been in the Word for a while, we suggest the Gospel of John, 1 John, Proverbs, or the Psalms because they are so rich with wisdom, praises, and obedience to God. However, be sensitive to the leading of the Lord in your reading. If He guides you somewhere else in the Bible, go there.

   • Jesus said it all in John 6:44,45: "No one can come to me unless the Father who sent me draws him, and I will raise him up at the last day. It is written in the Prophets: 'They will all be taught by God.' Everyone who listens to the Father and learns from him comes to me."

- Ultimately, it is God and His Holy Spirit who guide you and teach you.
- Food you eat is used up after three or four hours, and a twelve-hour antihistamine wears off after twelve hours. Spiritual feeding wears off after a few hours, too. You can't expect to get everything you need at Sunday morning service! You must return to Him frequently, but keep Him and His will in mind at all times. Attention to God takes our time—but He gives it back to us, plus some!

God made us as infants to be physically hungry about every three hours so that we would bond to our mothers and learn to depend on them for our needs. God has made us, as infant Christians, to be spiritually hungry probably every three hours or so. Notice that you will have no *"desire eating"* or as many yearnings for food if you will get your food from your Heavenly Father very frequently through praying or reading His Word. When you are in the desert and being tested, praying and reading will sometimes seem cold, icy, or dry. As time goes on and God transforms you, reading Scripture will be better than a pan of brownies! Hard to believe, but true!

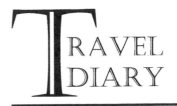

TRAVEL DIARY

Date I left Egypt: *June 20, 19--*

Loving thoughts to the Father

Lord, thank You for loving me the way You do. To go out last night and eat real Mexican food, chips and salsa — to stop with control. But most important, to feel Your acceptance. What peace! What freedom!

Heartfelt lessons from the Father

Lord, thank you for leading me to Ps. 81. It shows Your patience and love for me. It humbles and moves me to have you be so attentive to my desire to love You more. I cannot express how it feels to realize that You care about the smallest details. — letting me feel hunger, letting me taste the best and helping me stop at full. Loving You is fun.

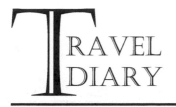

TRAVEL DIARY

Date:

Loving thoughts to the Father

_____
_____
_____
_____
_____
_____
_____
_____
_____
_____

Heartfelt lessons from the Father

_____
_____
_____
_____
_____
_____
_____
_____
_____
_____
_____

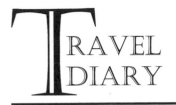

RAVEL
DIARY

Date: _____

Loving thoughts to the Father

_____
_____
_____
_____
_____
_____
_____
_____
_____
_____
_____

Heartfelt lessons from the Father

_____
_____
_____
_____
_____
_____
_____
_____
_____
_____
_____

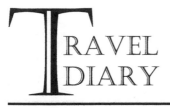

TRAVEL DIARY

Date:

Loving thoughts to the Father

Heartfelt lessons from the Father

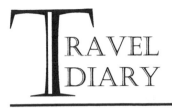

TRAVEL DIARY

Date: _____

Loving thoughts to the Father

_____
_____
_____
_____
_____
_____
_____
_____
_____
_____

Heartfelt lessons from the Father

_____
_____
_____
_____
_____
_____
_____
_____
_____
_____

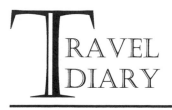

TRAVEL DIARY

Date: _____

Loving thoughts to the Father

_____

_____

_____

_____

_____

_____

_____

_____

_____

_____

_____

Heartfelt lessons from the Father

_____

_____

_____

_____

_____

_____

_____

_____

_____

_____

_____

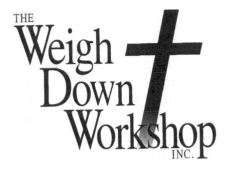

THE

Weigh Down Workshop
INC.

Imagine a person reporting that he ate only three-quarters of a burrito for the first time in his life and did not desire the rest of it. Imagine groups meeting together once a week and reporting the volume of their food intake decreasing but they feel happier than they have in years. Imagine people bringing in "before" pictures and sharing their weight loss of 100 pounds or more. Imagine groups of people from all backgrounds and denominations meeting together on one common ground . . . turning to God for strength. There are more than 30,000 such groups meeting worldwide and they are all part of The Weigh Down Workshop[t].

The Weigh Down Workshop[t] is a Bible-based seminar designed to teach people to distinguish between physical hunger and spiritual hunger, which frees them from thinking about food. It teaches people how to replace their relationship to food with a relationship to God, and many are experiencing permanent weight loss as a result.

In a series of twelve weekly classes, Weigh Down[t] participants watch videos that demonstrate the way thin eaters look, think, and behave. The host through these videos is Gwen Shamblin, R.D. Using her nutrition background and her strong Christ-centered approach, Gwen developed these materials that direct you to God for help in controlling bingeing and emotional eating. The sessions are casual and instructional in

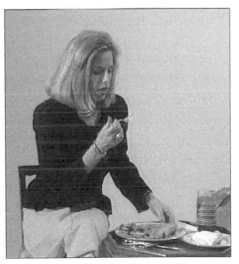

Class videos show you the behavior of thin eaters—people not magnetized toward food.

nature. They start with class videos that include testimonials from people who have lost 15–180 pounds, as well as from people who have overcome bulimia and anorexia. And all of this occurs without a diet, pills, or fat-gram counting. It is not religion, but it is a give-and-take relationship with God. "God did not put chocolate, sour cream, or blue cheese dressing down on earth to torture us," says Gwen. "Rather, God put them on earth for our enjoyment, and you can learn to eat them with control no matter how 'out of control' you feel!"

After the video, the remaining time is used for sharing and praying. There are no embarrassing weigh-ins. In contrast, you will hear how people have gone to God for help and how He has completely removed the desire to eat the second half of a meal. All forms of victory over emotional eating are shared, including weight loss, reduced stress, and a closer relationship with God.

The Weigh Down Workshop[†] presents revolutionary information. Many attempts are made in this day and age to make the environment change—making food lower in fat, taking pills, using liquid fasts, and doing "have-to" exercise routines. This weight-loss seminar is spreading rapidly because the workshop introduces *heart* modification. People are making the choice to love God in place of the refrigerator, resulting in dramatic changes in their lives.

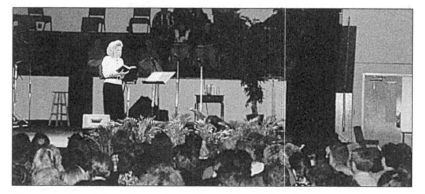

Thousands of people from all over the world meet in Nashville each summer for encouragement, songs of praise to God, and amazing testimonies.

If you are interested in a class location near you, please call, write, or fax the Weigh Down Workshop[†] at:

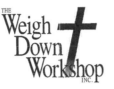

Weigh Down Workshop
P.O. Box 689099
Franklin, Tennessee 37068-9099
Phone: (800) 844-5208
Fax: (800) 340-2142

An Outreach Director will answer your phone call or letter and help you locate a class near you.

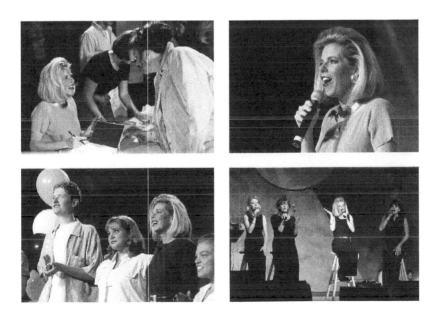